PCOS DIET COOKBOOK FOR BEGINNERS

500 Hormone Balancing Recipes to Relieve Symptoms

Ashley Adams

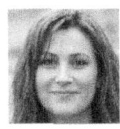

CONTENTS

Title Page
Copyright
Introduction
Recipes　3

Copyright © 2023 MyPCOSKitchen.com

All rights reserved

No part of this book may be reproduced, or stored in a retrieval system, or transmitted in any form or by any means, electronic, mechanical, photocopying, recording, or otherwise, without express written permission of the publisher.

INTRODUCTION

My Story

In 2010, I was officially diagnosed with PCOS, Polycystic Ovarian Syndrome. Doctors say that 1 in 10 women have it and more than 50% of women don't even know they have it.

The average woman sees at least 5 different practitioners before they even get a diagnosis. I myself dealt with at least 10 physicians before a doctor suggested I may have PCOS.

When I heard the news I thought to myself: Okay great. Now what? I didn't even know what PCOS meant, what it could do to the body, or that it would eventually get worse.

I asked the doctor what it was and the only thing she had told me was: well, do you have a boyfriend?

I told her no. She then told me that it wasn't really a big issue until I would be ready to have kids and until then she would just give me the pill so that my would come regularly.

That was the end of that. I took the pill and I fainted the first month. I decided to never take the pill again and ignored my symptoms. However, I find that the pill works differently on every one. For some women, it may regulate their period, for some it won't make them stop.

For me, my period came but made me extremely dizzy to the point where I fainted. At this time, I can't recommend the use of the pill because it doesn't fix the underlying problem, it just hides them.

At the time, ignoring my problems probably wasn't the best idea, but I had no idea what PCOS was and so didn't think too much of it.

After some time, my symptoms started getting worse and worse and I had no idea that they were all connected. The most common PCOS symptoms are as followed:

- Acne

- Hirsutism (facial hair)

- Irregular period, no period whatsoever, or period that will last literally months, non-stop

- Easy weight gain, obesity (especially in the abdominal area)

- Insulin resistance (dark patches on skin like the

back of you neck, underarms, between the breasts, groin area, on heels, etc)

- High cholesterol

- Thinning hair on scalp

- Infertility

- Many miscarriages

- Gluten Intolerance

- Ovarian cysts

- Diabetes

and the list goes on...

I have been personally struggling with irregular period hirsutism, obesity, insulin resistance, ovarian cysts, high cholesterol, pre-diabetes, and gluten intolerance. I first got my period when I was 11 years old, and they have been irregular since.

Doctors believed that they were irregular because I did a lot of exercise (gymnastics and cheerleading). My period were irregular in the sense that they would come on and off, or 6-10 times a year. However, when I turned 18 years old and moved out of my mom's house, different symptoms started to appear.

First was the weight gain. I had stopped doing sports

because I couldn't afford to go to a gymnastics gym and I was essentially on a student's budget. I bought the cheapest, easiest, most unhealthy food you could imagine and I started gaining weight. My friends used to tell me don't worry, it's normal.

It's called Frosh 15, where you gain 15 pounds the first year you move out. It'll be fine once you get used to living alone. Except that wasn't the case. That 15 pounds turned into 50 pounds, and I gained more weight every year.

My weight never went down and kept steadily going up. In 2010, I started getting hair on my face. I didn't know why this was happening to me. I'm a woman, I'm not supposed to have hair there. That's when I went to the doctor and she did an ultrasound of my ovaries.

After the diagnosis, I found out that I had multiple cysts on my ovaries and that I was insulin resistant. But that wasn't even the bad news. The bad news is that there is no known cure.

What does insulin resistance mean exactly? Well, insulin is a hormone that you make in your pancreas to control your blood sugar levels.

It acts mainly on fat and muscle cells, causing them to take in sugar when your blood sugar level rises; it also acts on the ovaries causing them to produce the male hormone testosterone.

Most women with PCOS have what is called insulin resistance, meaning that the cells in the body are resistant to the effect of normal level of insulin. More insulin is then produced to keep the blood sugar normal. T

his causes the ovaries to make too much testosterone, thus the facial hair, the thinning hair on scalps, and the irregular period.

Increased insulin also causes weight gain in the abdominal area because the overproduction of insulin turns into fat. Doctors believe that the underlying reason of PCOS is insulin resistance.

How I Cured My Hirsutism

The constant weight gain wasn't good for me. It isn't good for anybody. Because of it, my hirsutism became worse expanding everywhere on my face creating this "man beard".

It's embarrassing. No, it's humiliating. Having facial hair really hurt my self-confidence and self-esteem. I didn't have a boyfriend and I was too scared to approach guys that I had a crush on.

I had a male friend in university who asked me if I was a lesbian because I never had one-night stands or had a boyfriend...When people say stuff like that, it's really hard for someone to overcome it.

My self-confidence was as low as it could be. I decided to never approach guys again until I would regain my self-confidence and find a way to deal with my facial hair. You can read more about my facial hair on my blog: https://www.mypcoskitchen.com/pcos-facial-hair-electrolysis

While in university, most of my friends probably noticed that I had facial hair. I mean it was obvious. This facial hair is called hirsutism and is one of the most common symptoms of PCOS.

Because women with PCOS have insulin resistance, it causes the insulin to act on the ovaries and this causes them to produce male hormones, creating more testosterone.

This means that shaving, plucking, trimming, waxing, or bleaching will not, cannot, fix the problem. It only makes it worse.

I've seen hundreds of girls on PCOS forums posting that they didn't know what to do anymore because they have to shave twice a day and still see a five o'clock shadow 2 hours later. Some wives even joke that they have bigger beards than their husbands. At least they have a sense of humor.

My friends always told me to shave or wax my face. I did. Trust me. It only made it worse. The hair came out thicker, longer, and blacker than ever before.

Imagine having hair that is high on testosterone and hair that you've never had before suddenly appear in places you didn't know hair could exist! I plucked every day for hours and by the end of the day you could feel my prickly cheeks and chin.

In 2012, I decided to take all of my money and get laser hair removal. I had 8 painful treatments in 1 year and they all came back...triple the amount.

Not only did they all come back, but more of them started growing in spots I didn't use to have hair in.

The laser technologist then told me that electrolysis would probably be better a better option since electrolysis is the only real permanent option, whereas laser hair removal isn't.

Apparently, laser hair removal puts too much electric current and stress in your pores that it can cause an even bigger hormonal imbalance, stimulating the hair roots will cause those hormones to sort of fight back and make more hair, at least that's what an electrologist told me.

As a student, electrolysis was simply out of the question as it was far too expensive. I had wasted all of my money and my face had gotten worse. You can imagine how I felt.

Fixing Pcos The Natural Way

I think the hardest part of having PCOS are the people around you. They don't fully understand what is happening and try to give you advice that doesn't work like it would on a normal person.

I've had guy friends telling me to just lose weight, just don't eat for 2 days, just puke, just cut half my calories, and so on. These friends didn't understand that us ladies with PCOS fight these cravings every day.

We want to eat carbs and sugar, and to diet is extremely hard and takes a lot of self-control. We fight this urge every day. When someone has an illness, they can't just cure it like that.

It's like telling someone with Coeliac Disease to just take a pill and all of their symptoms will be gone, or that it's okay if you eat these gluten-free toast because they're made with gluten-free ingredients, except these toasts were toasted in a toaster that toasts normal bread and cross-contamination can make a person with CD so much sicker.

PCOS is a visible and invisible disorder that sometimes makes it hard for people to understand. It's not going to disappear in one day.

No, we have to work hard, much harder than a normal person, to make the symptoms lessen, but unfortunately, they will never fully disappear.

I gave up dealing with my facial hair while in

university, at least until I could find a job where I could afford electrolysis treatments every week. Starting in late 2014, I started researching more and more about PCOS and how it affects our bodies.

I finally understood that the more carbs I ate, the more my symptoms got worse. I basically had to start eating like a diabetic. A normal person's daily carb intake should be about 250g-350g, but eating that many carbs while dealing with PCOS makes everything worse.

I have found that the correct amount to eat and not have any symptoms is between 0-75g of carbs. The insulin levels in the blood go up after eating carbs meaning that your weight can increase, your hirsutism can go out of control, your cholesterol, blood sugar, and blood pressure all go up and it essentially can make your diabetic symptoms worsen.

It turns out that women with PCOS generally crave carbs. A lot of them. I can attest to that. It is so true.

I think the number one goal for women with PCOS should be to regulate their insulin levels. This can be fixed by medication that diabetic people use like Metformin, but I personally think that medication isn't always the best choice because it doesn't actually heal you, it just lessens some of your symptoms.

Metformin and other drugs have so many side effects, it's ridiculous. I think that eliminating as many carbs as you can will help regulate insulin, help you lose weight, and help balance those hormones.

I've never been good at doing diets, hell, I hate the word diet. That's why I started experimenting on various food and found that my body felt much better when I ate gluten-free and sugar-free. I've created two meal plans (7-day plan & 21-day plan) and have a long list of PCOS recipes on my site to help others get started. You can find those meal plans to download here:

- https://www.mypcoskitchen.com/pcos-7-day-meal-plan
- https://www.mypcoskitchen.com/21-day-keto-paleo-pcos-meal-plan

In July 2014, my mother and I decided to eat all organic to see if there would be any noticeable changes.

Well, surprise surprise. I got my period that month. Ever since I started gaining weight, my period came maybe 2-5 times a year if I were lucky. I never, I mean never, got them twice in a row. Sometimes they would only come once a year. Now, the first month we ate organic was in July 2014 and I got my period.

t could've been a coincidence so I waited until the next month. I got my period AGAIN. I ate organic in September too, and my period came again.

That was 3 months in a row where my period came

naturally and all I had to do was eat organic.

Unfortunately, I had just graduated from university and didn't have a job just yet and my mom didn't have lots of money so we had to quit the organic diet. Organic food can really add up.

I stopped eating organic at the end of September and my period also stopped coming. I randomly got them back in December 2014.

In January 2015, I got a job in Japan and moved there. In Japan, the food is made with much less pesticides and no growth hormones than the ones in North America or Europe.

To give you an example, eggs in N. America lasts a good 1-1.5 months. Here in Japan, they last about 10 days.

The vegetables you buy here rot much faster than the food back home. The meat I buy at the grocery is good for about 2 days and then it's rotten.

Back in Canada, I would always buy 2 weeks worth of groceries knowing the food will still be good, but during my first week in Japan, I bought 2 weeks worth of groceries and everything rotted 4-5 days later.

I always see pictures on Facebook of people meal prepping for the week where they prepare food and leave it in Tupperwares for 5 days.

I can't do that because 3 days in, the food starts to taste funny and you know it won't last 5. I've been living here since January 2015 and guess what? I have gotten my period every single month since.

I now definitely know that the poison they put in our food back home is making us sick. If I ever go back to Canada, I will ONLY eat organic.

I decided to only eat food grown in Japan, nothing from abroad, and only eat organic. I started a period tracker and I've been registering my basal body temperature every morning.

My period cycle alternate between 28 days to 34 days. I also ovulate every month . That is absolutely amazing, right? Just by changing what I ate, my period came back naturally without taking any medication.

(Period tracker: January 2014, July 2014, August 2014, September 2014, December 2014, February 2015-Present)

As for my hirsutism, with the new job that I have, I can finally afford to go get treatments.

I started my first treatments in March 2015 and went once a week for 45 minutes. In October 2015, I started going once a week but only for 30 minute sessions. In February 2016,

I started going 3 times a month instead of 4-5 and did 30 minute sessions. My hair has slowly been disappearing and my face is now normal. In June 2016, I started going once every 3 weeks, and in September 2016 I started alternating between once a month or once every 3 weeks.

In January 2018, I've been going once every 5 weeks. When I go, it's only to get the little persistent ones that keep on coming out. You cannot see any facial hair on my face right now as it is all clear.

The hairs that do grow back are short, light-coloured, and not thick. Their roots are also slowly disappearing. For your information, 5 hours costs about $650 CAD so it's not exactly cheap.

Electrolysis zaps one hair at a time with an electric current for 5-10 seconds, whereas laser hair removal can do your whole face in less than 5 minutes.

I was reading this website for trans-gendered people that went through electrolysis to get rid of their beards and it said that it usually takes 2-4 years of treatments to get rid of all the facial hair.

You first start with treatments every week (once or twice) and it eventually decreases to 1 treatment a month or every couple of months, to no more treatments at all. As long as I have a job, I will be continuing my electrolysis.

This has given me so much more confidence as a woman and I feel much better about myself.

As for my weight loss, I started to watch what I eat. I started to buy organic food from local farmers in February 2015.

I also started to watch my daily intake of carbs and try to limit myself to 75g of carbs a day or less. I don't really look at calories, just carbs. I stopped eating sugar and replaced it with stevia powder, erythritol and monk fruit powder.

I stopped eating gluten and have been trying different recipes using nuts and seeds flours. Living in Japan has been quite hard in finding different gluten-free versions of food because Japanese people are not accustomed to people with these kinds of dietary needs. Japan has a very carb-heavy diet.

They love bread, rice, deep-fried things, and put flour and sugar in literally everything. I allow myself one cheat day per week because if I didn't, I would quit right away and go back to eating unhealthy foods.

But on this cheat day, I don't necessarily eat gluten, more like I eat something that I've been craving like sushi. When I say sushi, I don't mean the sushi we serve back home, no, I mean Japanese style sushi.

Nigiri or sashimi to be exact.

The fish is much larger than the rice and there is nothing else like breadcrumbs and spicy mayo or random stuff you'll find back home.

I don't eat gluten or sugar at all. Not even on my cheat days. If I do eat something with gluten, I now get diarrhea and tummy aches which leads me to believe that I was actually gluten intolerant all this time.

A lot of sites suggest that women with PCOS should avoid eating dairy products. This is because dairy products contain the A1 casein which causes inflammation, which is not good for PCOS. But, having said that, not all cows produce this casein. Only Holstein cows do.

Jersey cows, goats and sheep produce the A2 casein which is fine for most people. I originally stopped eating dairy for about 4 months and didn't notice any difference.

I then ate dairy only from Jersey cows for about 6 months and again didn't notice any difference. That is why my recipes on my site still contain dairy. I'm always told that if you have PCOS, you're supposed to quit dairy, but I've never actually noticed or felt any different without dairy so I have not quit it.

I now eat regular dairy from any animals from time to time and I'm still losing weight and my health is still normal. So far, I haven't seen any reason to quit it. If it affects you negatively, then of couse, quit it. But for me, I was fine with it. I only use cream, yogurt and cheese.

I'm currently working on a "diet" plan that will

be totally organic, gluten-free, sugar-free, processed food-free, low-carb, low-calorie, sometimes paleo and that WILL involve meat, vegetables, fruits and dairy in moderation.

I would really love to eat lots of fruits, but unfortunately they are high in carbs AND they aren't really available in Japan. I mean they are, just ridiculously expensive. (For example, 1 small watermelon costs 10-50$). This is what my website is for.

I will upload all recipes that I know are extremely healthy for people with PCOS specifically, but also for people who follow a gluten-free lifestyle, paleo, ketogenic, or just want to lose weight, etc.

I have found that exercise also helps improve PCOS symptoms. I have to admit that before coming to Japan, I was in the worst shape of my life.

I remember in high school, I was in the gymnastics and cheerleading team, I could run for 5K and do unlimited amounts of conditioning. 1 year ago, I could barely run 100 meters.

I still have muscles and can manage about 50 sit-ups or 20 push-ups, but I would like to get my stamina back up.

Ever since I moved to Japan, I have been biking everywhere I go. I barely use the train, unless I go into Tokyo.

I bike to work, home, to the grocery, to my friend's house, etc. Back in Canada, I tried to bike for 10 minutes and I thought I was going to puke and pass out. I can proudly say that I can now bike 20km without taking a break.

I think that if I continue to bike everywhere and add a bit of conditioning here and there, that I will be able to lose weight in a healthy and safe way. I recommend to anyone with PCOS to do at least 20-30 minutes of exercise every day.

It honestly really does make a difference. I actually joined a gym and take their cardio kickboxing class every week! It doesn't really feel like exercise which is why I love it and I burn so much fat or calories with it!

So far, I have lost 95 pounds since March 2015 and I think that that is a healthy steady rate. My blood pressure is now normal 109/69, whereas it was 145/90 in December 2014.

My dark patches on my skin from the insulin resistance have completely disappeared. I am no longer pre-diabetic. My ultimate goal would be to lose 7 pounds a month, but we will see how that goes.

I would like to weigh 145 pounds as I think this is a healthy weight for a 5.4" female and want to try to reach that weight in the next 2 years.

My goal with this blog is to create recipes that are

mouth-watering, but that are also healthy and good for you.

Just because I crave a burger, doesn't mean that I should quit my diet. No, it only means that I have to create a healthy version that I will be able to enjoy 100% more.

Ever since I changed my lifestyle and my diet, I have felt more energized, less grumpy/cranky, felt more healthy, and I've been able to do more things that I couldn't do before.

I will continue living like this and continue to update my website whenever my body has changed. Thank you for reading this. PCOS isn't something I publicly talk about, but I feel that with my recipes that I have developed, I can help other cysters out there get healthy.

I'm not done losing weight and I still have a long way to go, but I know that I can do it, and if I can, so can you.

If you would like to read about my latest health update, you can check out my post here! I wrote a post about my progress after going for a check-up at the doctors! Hint: I was asked, are you sure you have PCOS?

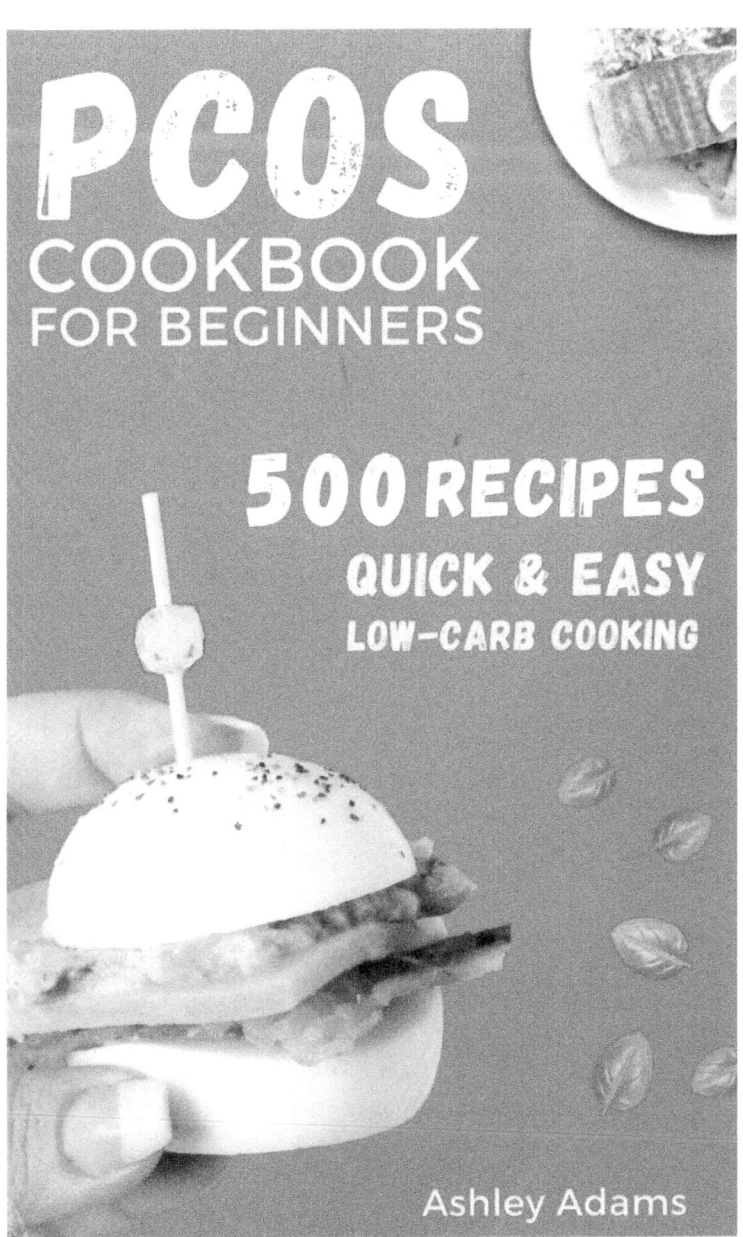

RECIPES

KETO PALEO GRANOLA

Ingredients:
- 1 cup cashews
- 3/4 cup almonds
- 1/4 cup pumpkin seeds
- 1/4 cup sunflower seeds
- 1/2 cup unsweetened coconut flakes
- 1/4 cup coconut oil
- Stevia to taste
- 1 tsp vanilla

Instructions:
- Preheat the oven to 300 degrees F. Line a baking sheet with parchment paper.

- Place the cashews, almonds, coconut flakes and pumpkin seeds into a blender and pulse to break the mixture into smaller pieces.

- In a large microwave-safe bowl, melt the coconut oil, vanilla, and stevia together for 40-50 seconds.

Add in the mixture from the blender and the sunflower seeds, and stir to coat.

- Spread the mixture out onto the baking sheet and cook for 20-25 minutes, stirring once, until the mixture is lightly browned. Remove from heat.

- Press the granola mixture together to form a flat, even surface. Cool for about 15 minutes, and then break into chunks.

CHICKEN PATTIES

Ingredients:

- 2 cups cooked ground chicken meat
- 2 large eggs
- 1 tsp of salt
- 1 tsp of garlic powder
- 1 tsp dried chopped onion
- 1/2 tsp of pepper
- 1/2 tsp smoked paprika
- 1 cup grated Parmesan cheese
- 1/2 cup finely chopped and cooked spinach
- 2 tbsp finely chopped parsley
- Pork rinds

Instructions:

- Combine cooked chicken, salt, garlic powder, minced onion, pepper, smoked paprika, Parmesan cheese, spinach, and parsley in a large mixing bowl.

- Pack firmly and form into equal-sized patties. Place patties in the freezer for 15 to 20 minutes until they begin to firm up.

- Whisk egg in a medium bowl. Place chopped pork rind and dill in a large bowl.

- Dip each chicken patty into the egg, then press it into the pork rind to coat. Place them in the basket of the air fryer.

- Set the temperature to 360°F and set the timer for 12 minutes.

SHRIMP COATED WITH COCONUT

Ingredients:
- 1 lb shrimp with tails
- 1 beaten egg
- 1 cup shredded coconut
- 1 tsp garlic powder
- 1 tsp paprika
- 1 tsp onion powder
- 1 tsp salt

Instructions:

- Place the shredded coconut in a bowl with the garlic powder, paprika, onion powder, and salt, then beat the egg in another bowl.

- Use a cooking oil spray to coat the bottom of the air fryer basket. Then place a shrimp in the bowl with the beaten egg and coat it.

- Transfer it to the bowl with the shredded coconut and coat. Immediately place the coconut shrimp in the fryer basket.

- Repeat step 3 until the air fryer basket is filled with shrimp in a single layer.
- Cook at 350 degrees for 10 minutes. Remove the shrimps and serve with your favorite sauce.

PROTEIN MUESLI

Ingredients:
- 1 cup unsweetened coconut flakes
- 1 tbsp chopped walnuts
- 1 tbsp raw almonds
- 1 tbsp chocolate chips
- 1/2 tsp cinnamon
- 1 cup unsweetened almond milk
- 1 scoop hemp protein

Instructions:
- In a medium bowl layer coconut flakes, walnuts, almonds, and chocolate chips.
- Sprinkle with cinnamon. Pour cold almond milk over the muesli and enjoy.

NUTTY GRANOLA

Ingredients:
- 1 cup of coconut milk
- 1 tsp of pecan pieces
- 1 tsp of walnut pieces

- 1 tsp of slivered almonds
- 1 tsp of unsalted pistachio
- 1 tsp of pine nuts
- 1 tsp of sunflower seeds
- 1 tsp raw pumpkin seeds
- 2 tbsp of frozen or fresh berries

Instructions:
- Put all the nuts & seeds in a bowl.

- Add the berries and milk. If using frozen berries, wait for 2-3 minutes for them to get warmer. Enjoy!

PARMESAN & LEMON ASPARAGUS

Ingredients:
- 1 bunch of asparagus
- 1 teaspoon of olive oil
- 1/8 teaspoon garlic salt
- 1 tablespoon grated Parmesan cheese
- Black pepper to taste
- 1 tablespoon lemon juice

Instructions:
- Clean asparagus and dry. Cut the bottom off to remove woody sprigs.

- Place asparagus in a single layer in the air fryer and drizzle with oil and lemon juice.

- Sprinkle the garlic salt equally across the tops of the asparagus. Season with pepper and add a little Parmesan cheese.

- Bake at 400 degrees for 7 - 10 minutes.

- After removing the asparagus from the air fryer, add a little Parmesan cheese on top.

APPLE ALMOND MEDLEY

Ingredients:

- 1/2 apple cored and diced
- A handful of sliced almonds
- A handful of unsweetened coconut
- A pinch of cinnamon
- 1 pinch of salt

Instructions:

- Pulse in the food processor to desired consistency.
- Serve with almond milk, or coconut milk.

CHOCOLATE NUT MUESLI BALLS

Ingredients:

- 1 cup of raw almonds
- 1 Tablespoon of coconut oil
- 2 Tablespoon Coconut flour
- 1 egg white
- 2 Tablespoon + 1 teaspoon of Cacao powder
- 1/2 cup of liquid stevia

Instructions:

- First, grind the almonds in a food processor or blender until you have a flour.

- Add the ground almonds, coconut flour, egg white, liquid stevia and cacao powder to a bowl and mix with a spoon until you have a dough.

- Take a small pinch of the dough and roll into a round ball and set on a baking sheet lined with parchment paper.

- Turn on your oven and set to 350 degrees and bake for 15 minutes.

- Remove from the oven and let cool on the pan. Top with your favorite milk and enjoy!

LIGHT CRACKERS

Ingredients:

- 1 egg
- liquid stevia to taste
- 1 Tbsp coconut oil
- 1 1/2 cups almond flour
- 5 cup coconut flour
- 1 teaspoon cinnamon

Instructions:

- Preheat the oven to 350 F. In a large bowl, whisk together the egg, pure liquid stevia and melted coconut oil.

- Add the coconut and almond flour and stir to combine.

- Give the dough a couple of kneads so it's well incorporated.

- Turn the dough onto a piece of parchment paper and flatten a bit with your hands.

- Place another piece of parchment on top and roll out with a rolling pin until it's about 1/8 inch thick.

- Remove the top piece of parchment and cut the dough into 1/4 inch squares.

- Sprinkle the cinnamon into the dough mixture.

- Slide the dough with the bottom parchment paper onto a baking sheet and bake for 15 minutes.

- Turn down the oven to 325 F and bake for another 10-15 minutes.

VEGGIE BREAKFAST PEPPERS

Ingredients:
- 2 bell peppers
- 4 eggs
- 1 cup white mushrooms
- 1 cup broccoli
- 1/2 tsp cayenne pepper
- low sodium salt and pepper, to taste

Instructions:
- Preheat the oven to 375 degrees Fahrenheit.

- Dice up your vegetables of choice.

- In a medium sized bowl, mix eggs, low sodium salt, pepper, cayenne pepper, and vegetables.

- Cut peppers into equal halves.

- Core the peppers so that they're clean enough to add the filling.

- Pour a quarter of the egg / vegetable mixture into each pepper halve, adding more vegetables to the top to fill in any empty space.

- Place on a baking sheet and cook for approximately 35 minutes.

BREAKFAST MEXICANA

Ingredients:

For the tortillas:
- 2 eggs
- 2 egg whites
- 1/2 cup water
- 4 tsp ground flax-seed
- Pinch of salt

For the filling:
- 1 avocado, diced
- 1/4 cup red bell
- pepper, finely diced
- 1/4 cup onion, finely diced
- 1/4 cup baked cod or other protein
- Handful of spinach leaves
- 1 tsp coconut oil

Instructions:

- In a small bowl, whisk together the ingredients for the tortilla. Preheat the oven.

- Heat a 10-inch non-stick skillet over medium heat and coat well with coconut oil spray.

- Pour half of the tortilla mixture into the pan and swirl to evenly distribute. Using a metal spatula, loosen the edges of the tortilla from the pan.

- Cook for a couple of minutes until golden brown on the bottom, and then carefully slide the spatula under the tortilla to loosen it from the bottom of the pan. Do not flip yet.

- Place the pan under the broiler for 3-4 minutes until the tortilla gets a little bubbly.

- Remove the tortilla from the pan, setting on a piece of aluminum foil. Repeat with the other half of the tortilla mixture.

- After the tortillas are done broiling, preheat the oven to 400 degrees F.

- In a separate small pan, heat the coconut oil over medium heat. Add the onions and peppers and saute for 5-8 minutes, until soft. Add the spinach into the pan and wilt.

- Place all of the fillings down the center of the tortillas and wrap tightly. Place into the oven for 5-8 minutes to set.

VEGETARIAN CURRY WITH SQUASH

Ingredients:

- 1 tbsp coconut oil
- 2 cups mixed raw nuts
- 1 medium yellow onion, diced
- 1 tsp low sodium salt
- 1 green bell pepper, thinly sliced
- 4 cloves garlic, minced
- 1-inch piece fresh ginger, peeled and minced
- 1 14-oz. can coconut milk
- 1 large acorn squash, peeled, seeded, and cut into 1-inch cubes
- 2 tsp lime juice
- 1 teaspoon curry powder (mild or hot)
- 1/4 cup cilantro, chopped
- Cauliflower rice, for serving

Instructions:

- Melt the coconut oil in a large pan over medium heat. Add the onion and cook for 5-6 minutes, stirring occasionally. Add the bell pepper, garlic, ginger, and low sodium salt and stir to combine. Cook for an additional minute.

- Add the curry powder to the pan and cook for about a minute, stirring to coat the other ingredients. Add in the coconut milk and bring to a simmer. Stir in the squash.

- Simmer, stirring occasionally, for 15-20 minutes until the squash is fork- tender. Remove the pan from the heat and stir in the lime juice. Taste and adjust low sodium salt and lime juice as necessary. Sprinkle with cilantro to serve.

- Roast the nuts under the grill until crisp and sprinkle over the top of the curry.

SAUCY GRATIN WITH CREAMY CAULIFLOWER BONANZA

Ingredients:
- 1 medium butternut squash, peeled, seeded, and diced
- 1 large sweet potato, peeled and thinly sliced
- 6 cups fresh spinach
- 1 tbsp extra virgin olive oil
- 2 large shallots, diced
- 4 cloves garlic, chopped
- salt and pepper, to taste
- Pinch of nutmeg

For the sauce:
- 1/2 head of cauliflower, cut into florets
- 1 cup almond milk
- 1/2 cup low sodium chicken stock
- 1/2 tsp low sodium salt
- 1/2 tsp freshly ground pepper
- 1/4 tsp nutmeg

Instructions:
- Preheat the oven to 375 degrees F. To make the cream sauce, place a couple inches of water in a large pot. Once the water is boiling, place a steamer

and then cauliflower florets into the pot and cover. Steam for 12-14 minutes, until completely tender.

- Drain and return cauliflower to the pot. Add the almond milk, stock, nutmeg, low sodium salt, and pepper to the pot. Use an immersion blender or food processor to combine the ingredients until smooth. Set aside. Meanwhile, bring a separate pot of water to a boil. Add the butternut squash and cook for 4 minutes. Drain and set aside.

- Heat the oil in a small pan over medium heat. Add the shallots and garlic and cook for 4-5 minutes until soft. Stir in the spinach to wilt. Season with low sodium salt and pepper.

- To assemble, grease a large baking dish with coconut oil spray. Spoon a thin layer of the cream sauce over the bottom of the pan.

- Arrange a layer of half of the butternut squash. Top with half of the spinach mixture, and then all of the sliced sweet potato.

- Drizzle with the cream sauce. Add the remaining half of the spinach, followed by the rest of the butternut squash. Drizzle the rest of the cream sauce over the top.

- Sprinkle with low sodium salt, pepper, and nutmeg. Bake for 50-60 minutes until browned. Allow to cool for 10 minutes.
E
GG BOK CHOY AND BASIL STIR-FRY

Ingredients:
- 1 tablespoon fish sauce
- 1 garlic clove, minced
- 3 eggs
- 2 tablespoons olive oil
- 1 small onion, finely chopped
- 1-inch piece fresh ginger, chopped
- 2 red chilies, thinly sliced crosswise
- 1 cup thinly sliced bok choy stems
- 1 cup thinly sliced bok choy greens
- handful fresh basil leaves, chopped
- juice of 1 lime

Instructions:
- In a large bowl mix fish sauce, garlic and ginger.

- Heat the olive oil in a wok (or a large nonstick skillet) over medium-high heat. Once it starts to shimmer add onion and chilies. Stir-fry the onions until they start to brown around the edges, about 2 minutes.

- Stir in the bok choy stems and stir-fry for 1 minute.

- Add the beaten eggs and cook until it's nearly cooked through about 2 minutes, stirring often.

- Stir in bok choy greens, basil and lime juice. And stir-fry for 30 seconds or so, until the greens are wilted. Serve immediately.

EGG VEGETABLE STIR FRY

Ingredients:
- 1 lb of Cubed Butternut Squash
- 1 lb of Green Beans
- 3 Baby Bok Choys
- 1lb of Eggplants
- 3 Garlic Cloves
- 1 small onion
- 1 tsp of salt
- 1 tsp of Black Pepper
- 1-2 tbsp of coconut oil
- 3 eggs

Instructions:
- Peel, core, and cut the butternut squash into 1" cubes.

- Snap the ends off the green beans and slice at an angle into 1.5" long pieces.

- Chop the bok choy leaves from the stems. Slice the stems into 1" thick pieces. Cut the leaves in half.

- Slice the eggplants into 1" thick discs, then quarter the disc into wedges. Slice in half if the eggplant is skinny.

- Mince the garlic cloves and slice the onions. Heat a wok and add the cooking oil.

- Add the onions and cook until translucent. About 2 minutes. Add the garlic and cook for another minute.

- Add the squash, beans, low salt, and pepper.

Add the eggplant and bok choy stalks and cook uncovered for another 7- 10 minutes.

- Add the bok choy leaves and cook for another few minutes, covered.

- Beat the eggs and add them to the stir fry, and keep stirring till they are cooked through

ARUGULA SALAD

Ingredients:
- 4 tsp fresh lemon juice
- 4 tsp walnut oil
- salt and freshly ground pepper
- 6 cups arugula leaves
- Garlic powder to taste

Instructions:
- Pour the lemon juice into a large bowl. Gradually whisk in the oil. Season with salt and pepper.

- Add the greens, toss until evenly dressed and serve at once. Feel free to add tomatoes or grated carrot and onion slices.

SPRING SALAD

Ingredients:
- 5 cups of salad greens of choice

Dressing:
- 1/2 cup olive oil
- 3 tbsp lemon juice
- 1 tbsp mustard powder
- salt
- Black pepper

Instructions:
- Combine salad greens and any other raw vegetables of choice.

- Combine oil, lemon juice and mustard. Mix well.

- Add salt and pepper to taste.

- Pour dressing over salad, toss and serve.

SPINACH & POMEGRANATE SALAD

Ingredients:
- 1 small bunch fresh spinach
- 12 dandelion leaves
- 1 cup pomegranate seeds
- 1/2 cup pecan halves

Instructions:
- You may substitute appropriate fresh greens for the dandelion and sorrel leaves.

- Wash and destem spinach. Pick and wash sorrel and dandelions.

- Coarsely chop dandelion leaves, and tear spinach, then toss dandelion, sorrel and spinach together in a stainless steel bowl. Put aside in the refrigerator to drain and cool.

- When drained, pour off excess water, and add pomegranate and pecans. Toss with dressing and serve.

CHICKEN SALAD

Ingredients:
- 1 Cooked and chopped chicken breast

- 1/4 cup Chopped almonds
- 1 Mashed avocado
- salt and pepper
- Any lettuce leaves of choice

   Instructions:
- Mix the first six ingredients together in a bowl.

- Season with salt and pepper, and then spoon onto lettuce leaves.

- Roll up and enjoy!

AVOCADO TUNA SALAD

   Ingredients:
- 2 tins of tuna
- 1 avocado
- 1/4 of an onion, chopped
- juice of 1/2 a lime
- 2 Tbsp cilantro
- salt and pepper to taste

   Instructions:
- Shred the tuna.
- Add all of the other ingredients and mix.

MACADAMIA TURKEY SALAD

Ingredients:

- 1 lb turkey breast
- 1 tsp nut oil
- salt and pepper
- 1/2 cup chopped macadamia nuts
- 1/2 cup diced celery
- 3 tbsp divine dressing
- 2 tbsp julienned basil
- 1 tbsp lemon juice

Instructions:

Divine Dressing:

- Mix together, 4 Tbsp. chili powder, 1 tsp each garlic powder, onion powder, and oregano, 2 tsp each paprika and cumin, 4 tsp low sodium salt, and 1/8 1/4 tsp red pepper flakes. Add 1 cup olive oil and half cup rice vinegar.

- Preheat the oven to 350 degrees. Place chicken breasts on a sheet tray, drizzle with oil, salt and pepper.

- Bake for about 35 minutes until cooked through. Remove from the oven and let cool.

- In a large bowl shred chicken. Add nuts, celery, basil, mayo, lemon juice, salt and pepper, dressing. Gently stir until combined.

RED CABBAGE SALAD

Ingredients:

For the chicken:
- 1/2 lb chicken mince
- 1 long red chili, finely chopped with the seeds
- 2 garlic cloves, finely chopped
- Little knob of fresh ginger, peeled and finely chopped
- 1 stem lemon grass, pale section only, finely chopped
- 1/2 bunch of coriander stems washed and chopped
- 1 tbsp low sodium salt
- 1 tbsp coconut aminos
- 1/2 lime rind grated
- 1/2 lime, juiced
- A pinch of low sodium salt
- Coconut oil for frying

For the salad:

- 1/4 red cabbage, thinly sliced
- 1 large carrot, peeled and grated
- 1/2 Spanish onion, thinly sliced
- 2 tbsp green spring onion, chopped
- 1/2 bunch of fresh coriander leaves
- A handful of fresh mint
- 1/2 cup crushed roasted cashews or some sesame seeds

For the dressing:
- 2 tbsp olive oil
- 3 tbsp lime juice
- 1 small red chili, finely chopped

Instructions:

- Heat 1 tbsp of coconut oil in a large frying pan. Throw in lemongrass, chili, garlic, coriander stems and ginger and stir fry for about a minute until fragrant.

- Add chicken mince and lime zest. Stir and break apart the mince with a wooden mixing spoon until separated into small pieces.

- The meat will now be changing to white color. Add lime juice. Stir through and cook for a further few minutes. Total cooking time for the chicken should be about 10 minutes.

- Prepare the salad base by mixing together sliced red cabbage, onion grated carrot, and fresh herbs.

- Mix all dressing ingredients and toss through the salad.

- Serve cooked chicken mince on top of the dressed salad and topped with roasted cashews, dried shallots, coconut flakes and extra fresh herbs.

SPROUTS SALAD

Ingredients:

- 1/2 lb of mixed sprouts
- 1/2 Granny Smith apple
- 1/2 cup chopped almonds
- 2 chicken breasts, chopped
- 1/2 white onion, finely diced

Vinaigrette:

- 2 tbsp Apple Cider Vinegar
- 1 tbsp brown mustard
- 1 tbsp avocado oil
- Stevia to taste
- 1/2 tsp salt
- black pepper

Instructions:

- Cut Granny Smith apple, slicing into matchsticks. Chop the half cup of almonds. Finely dice the white onion.

- Remove the breasts and chop into bite-sized pieces. Combine all of these ingredients into a large bowl and gently toss the sprouts into the salad.

- Whipping up the vinaigrette takes seconds. Add all ingredients to a small bowl and whisk until smooth. Pour over the sprouts salad and toss to bring together.

AVOCADO EGG SALAD

Ingredients:
- 1/4 cup Chopped almonds
- 3 cooked and chopped eggs
- 1 Mashed avocado
- salt and pepper
- lettuce leaves

Instructions:

- Mix the ingredients together in a bowl, season with salt and pepper, and then spoon onto lettuce leaves.

- Roll up and enjoy!

AVOCADO SALAD

Ingredients:
- 1 lb boneless, skinless chicken breasts
- 1 avocado
- 1/4 of an onion, chopped
- juice of 1 lime and 1 lemon

- 2 tbsp cilantro
- salt and pepper to taste
- 1 bag mixed lettuce leaves
- 1 tbsp olive oil

Instructions:

- Cook chicken breast until done, let cool, and then shred.

- Add all of the other ingredients and mix.

CLASSIC WALDORF SALAD

Ingredients:

- 2 lbs cooked chicken
- 1/2 cup onion, chopped
- 2-3 stalks celery, chopped
- 1/2 cup pecans, chopped (optional)
- 1 large apple
- 1/2 tsp salt
- 1/2 tsp Lemon Garlic
- Black pepper to taste
- 1 tbsp lemon juice
- Divine dressing

Instructions:

- First cook up a whole chicken. You can buy a rotisserie chicken, or throw a chicken in the crock pot, sprinkle it with cumin, low sodium salt & pepper and let it cook for about 4-6 hours on low.

- After the chicken is cooked and cooled, de-bone and shred the meat and put it in a large mixing bowl.

- Then do a bunch of chopping. Peel your apple, then chop your apple, onions, celery, and pecans.

- Combine all of these ingredients in the bowl with your chicken and then start adding the dressing. You will need enough to cover all the ingredients and make them moist, but not overly runny or dry.

- Add the low sodium salt and pepper, and lemon juice. Stir well to combine.

CLASSIC TUNA SALAD

Ingredients:
- 2 large grilled tuna steaks
- 2 tablespoons olive oil
- 1/2 cup onion, chopped
- 2-3 stalks celery, chopped
- Salt to taste
- 1 tsp Lemon Garlic pepper
- 1 Tbsp lemon juice

Instructions:
- Grill the tuna steaks medium rare with garlic powder and black pepper to taste.

- Combine all of these ingredients

in the bowl with your cubed tuna and then start adding the dressing of oil and lemon juice seasoned.

- You want enough to cover all the ingredients and make them moist, but not overly runny or dry. It tastes great served right away, but even better after it sits in the fridge for a day.

ARTICHOKE TUNA DELIGHT

Ingredients:
- 1 1/2 cups diced grilled tuna
- 1 cup finely diced red onion
- 1 small carrot julienned and cut into small pieces
- 4-5 artichoke hearts ; diced
- 2 tbsp capers
- salt and pepper to taste.
- 6 Radicchio leaves

Instructions:
- Place all ingredients, except the radicchio leaves in a large bowl and combine.

- Place a scoop of salad into each Radicchio cup and serve.

TUNA STUFFED TOMATO

Ingredients:
- 2 large tomatoes
- Lettuce leaves (optional)
- 2 6 oz cans tuna
- 6 Tbsp olive oil
- 1 tablespoon rice vinegar
- 1 stalk celery, chopped
- 1/2 small onion, chopped
- 1/4 tsp salt
- 1/4 ts. ground black pepper

Instructions:

- Wash and dry the tomatoes and remove any stem. You can either slice off the top part of the tomatoes and hollow them out, or cut each tomato into wedges, making sure to only cut down to about 1/2 inch before you get to the bottom of the tomato.

- Arrange the tomatoes on a plate on top of lettuce leaves (optional).

- Combine the remaining ingredients in a mixing bowl and add additional salt and/or pepper if desired. Spoon into the tomatoes and serve.

AVOCADO TUNA SALAD

Ingredients:
- 1 avocado
- 1 lemon, juiced
- 1 tablespoon chopped onion
- 1 cup chopped tomatoes
- 5 oz canned wild tuna
- low sodium salt and pepper to taste

Instructions:
- Cut the avocado in half and scoop the middle of both avocado halves into
a bowl, leaving a shell of avocado flesh about 1/4-inch thick on each half.

- Add lemon juice and onion to the avocado in the bowl and mash together.

- Add tuna, low sodium salt and pepper, and stir to combine. Taste and adjust if needed.

- Fill avocado shells with tuna salad and serve.

ITALIAN TUNA SALAD

Ingredients:
- 10 sun-dried tomatoes
- 2 (5 oz) can of tuna
- 1-2 ribs of celery, diced finely
- 2 tbsp of extra virgin olive oil
- 1 cloves garlic, minced
- 3 tbsp finely chopped parsley
- 1/2 tbsp lemon juice
- salt and pepper to taste

Instructions:

- Prepare the sun-dried tomatoes by softening them in warm water for 30 minutes until soft. Then, pat the tomatoes dry and chop finely.

- Flake the tuna. Mix the tuna together with the chopped tomatoes, celery, extra virgin olive oil, garlic, parsley, and lemon juice. Add low sodium salt and pepper to taste.

- If not served immediately, mix with extra olive oil just before serving.

TURKEY BOK CHOY SALAD

Ingredients:

For the salad:
- 2 cups grilled turkey, chopped
- 6 baby bok choy, grilled & chopped
- 2 green onions, chopped
- 1/4 cup cilantro, chopped
- 1 Tbsp sesame seeds

For the dressing:
- 1 Tbsp fresh ginger, chopped
- 2 Tbsp coconut cream
- 1 Tbsp soy sauce
- 1 Tbsp sesame oil
- 2 Tbsp fresh lime juice
- 1 Tbsp stevia powder

Instructions:

- Combine all of the salad ingredients until well mixed.

- Add all of the ingredients for the dressing into a blender or food processor, and blend until mostly smooth

- Pour the dressing over the salad and toss lightly until coated.

- Garnish with more sesame seeds if desired.

MEDITERRANEAN SALAD

Ingredients:

- 1 roasted chicken

Dressing:
  - 1/2 cup apple cider vinegar
  - garlic & onion powder to taste
  - 1/2 cup olive oil

Salad:
  - 1/4 cup fresh cilantro, chopped
  - 1 head of romaine or butter lettuce
  - 1 red onion, diced
  - 1 lemon, juiced
  - salt and pepper to taste

Instructions:

- Shred the chicken or chop up and put it in a big bowl.

- Add the dressing, red onion, cilantro, lemon, salt & pepper.

- Mix well and serve on a lettuce boat.

SPICY EASTERN SALAD

Ingredients:
- 2/3 cup fresh lime juice
- 1/3 cup fish sauce(optional)
- Stevia to taste
- 3/4 cup low sodium chicken stock
- 1 1/2 pounds ground chicken or turkey
- 1 cup thinly sliced green onions
- 3/4 cup thinly sliced shallots
- 3 tablespoons minced lemongrass
- 1 tablespoon thinly sliced Serrano chili
- 1/2 cup chopped cilantro leaves
- 1/3 cup chopped mint leaves
- salt
- 1 head of lettuce

Instructions:

- Whisk together lime juice, fish sauce ,stevia and Set aside.

- Warm chicken stock in a medium heavy-bottomed pot over medium heat until simmering.

- Add ground chicken and simmer until cooked through. As the chicken is cooking, stir occasionally to break up the meat. This should take 6 to 8 minutes.

- Add green onion, shallot, lemongrass and chilies, stirring to combine. Continue cooking until shallots turn translucent, stirring occasionally (about 4 minutes).

- Remove from the heat and drain off any liquid in the pot.

- Stir in lime juice-fish sauce mixture, cilantro and mint. Season to taste with low sodium salt.

- Transfer mixture to a large bowl and serve beside a pile of lettuce leaves. Using a slotted spoon, scoop on the lettuce leaves and enjoy!

LEMON TILAPIA

Ingredients:
- 6 tilapia filets
- 4 cloves garlic, crushed
- 2 tbsp olive oil
- 2 tbsp fresh lemon juice
- 4 tsp fresh parsley
- salt and pepper to taste
- 1 large romaine lettuce
- 1 grated carrot
- 1/2 grated onion
- handful baby spinach
- 2 tomatoes

Paleo Dressing:
- 2 tbsp best quality olive oil
- 1 tbsp apple cider vinegar
- 1 tbsp lemon juice

- 1/2 tsp garlic powder and half teaspoon onion powder
- Black pepper to taste

Instructions:

- Preheat the oven to 400°F. Melt butter on a low flame in a small saucepan. Add garlic and saute on low for about 1 minute. Add the lemon juice and shut off the flame.

- Spray the bottom of a baking dish lightly with cooking spray. Place the fish on top and season with salt and pepper. Pour the lemon butter mixture on the fish and top with fresh parsley.

- Bake for about 15 minutes. Serve with a mixed salad and paleo dressing.

PRAWN SKEWERS

Ingredients:

- 1 lb jumbo raw tiger prawns, shelled and deveined
- 2 cloves garlic, crushed
- salt and pepper

Instructions:

- Soak the skewers in water for at least 20 minutes to prevent them from burning. Combine the prawns with crushed garlic and season with low sodium salt and pepper. You can let this marinate for a while, or even overnight.

- Heat a clean, lightly oiled grill to medium

heat, when the grill is hot add the prawns, careful not to burn the skewers. Grill on both sides for about 6 - 8 minutes total cooking time or until the prawns are opaque and cooked through.

- Squeeze lemon juice over the prawns and serve with green salad and paleo dressing

SEARED SALMON WITH PEACH SALSA

Ingredients:

For the peach salsa:

- 1 large ripe peach peeled, seeded and coarsely chopped
- 1-2 tbsp chopped fresh cilantro
- 1 small clove garlic, minced
- 2 tbsp fresh lime juice

For the salmon:

- 1 tbsp paprika
- 1 tbsp cayenne
- 5 sprigs fresh thyme, w ashed, leaves removed and chopped
- 1 tbsp freshly chopped oregano leaves
- 1 tsp salt
- 1 lb wild salmon filet, skin-on

Instructions:

- Combine all the salsa ingredients in a bowl, season to taste with low sodium salt and pepper and refrigerate salsa until ready to serve.

- In a small bowl, add the paprika, cayenne,

thyme and oregano and low sodium salt and mix to blend. Put the mixture on a plate or other flat surface and coat the salmon filets.

- Heat a large heavy-bottomed pan or cast iron skillet over medium heat, and generously spray with oil. When very hot add the salmon, flesh side down and cook for 2 to 3 minutes. Use a spatula to carefully turn the salmon, then cook for an additional 5 to 6 minutes.

- Arrange the salmon on a platter, top with salsa and serve immediately with a green salad.

ROSEMARY SALMON

Ingredients:
- 4 pieces of salmon
- olive oil spray
- 2 tsp fresh lemon juice
- 2 tsp fresh, chopped rosemary
- 2 cloves garlic, minced
- salt and fresh pepper to taste

Instructions:

- Combine lemon juice, rosemary, low sodium salt, pepper and garlic. Brush mixture onto fish.

- Spray a ridged frying pan with olive oil spray and arrange the fish on it.

- Cook to level of preferred inner pinkness!...and turn of course

CURRY COCONUT COD

Ingredients:
- 1 tsp dark sesame oil, divided
- 1 tbsp minced peeled fresh ginger
- 4 garlic cloves, minced
- 1 cup finely chopped red bell pepper
- 1 cup chopped scallions
- 1 tsp curry powder
- 2 tsp red curry paste
- 1/2 tsp ground cumin
- 4 tsp low-sodium soy sauce
- Stevia to taste
- 14 oz can light coconut milk
- 1/4 cup chopped fresh cilantro
- 6 cod filets
- salt

Instructions:

- Preheat broiler. Heat 1/2 teaspoon oil in a large nonstick skillet over medium heat. Add ginger and garlic; cook for 1 minute. Add pepper and scallions; cook for 1 minute. Stir in curry powder, curry paste, and cumin; cook for 1 minute.

- Add soy sauce, stevia, and coconut milk; bring to a simmer (do not boil). Remove from heat; stir in cilantro or basil if using.

- Brush fish with 1/2 teaspoon oil; sprinkle with 1/4 teaspoon low sodium salt. Place fish on a baking sheet coated with cooking spray. Broil 7 minutes or until fish flakes easily when tested with a fork.

SHRIMP ON STICKS

Ingredients:
- 1/2 lb shrimp, peeled and deveined
- 1/4 cup coconut milk
- 1 tsp fish sauce
- 6 cloves garlic, chopped
- 1/4 tsp each turmeric, cumin, low sodium salt

Instructions:

- Heat olive oil in a large pan over medium heat. Add onion and garlic and cook until tender. Add chili flakes and stir for about a minute.

- When that has cooked down, add the diced tomatoes and oregano. Simmer for about 10 minutes.

- Add julienned zucchini and lemon juice and cook, stirring, for about 5 minutes.

- Add shrimp and then the spinach, once shrimp is just cooked through. Low sodium salt and pepper to taste and serve with a fresh squeeze of lemon.

FISH STIR FRY

Ingredients:

- 1 tbsp Coconut Vinegar
- 7 oz white fish filet into pieces
- 1/2 tsp Ginger and Garlic freshly pressed
- 1 small onion (quartered)
- 1/2 Cup Bell Peppers de-seeded and cubed (Red or Yellow).
- 1/2 Cup Mushrooms
- 2 to 3 stalks of scallions
- salt to taste
- 1 tsp Chili powder (Optional)
- 1 tsp Fish Sauce

Instructions:

- Heat 2 tbsp. coconut oil in a wok or large pan. Add the sliced garlic and grated ginger to the wok and stir-fry for 30 seconds.

- Add the scallions and stir-fry 1 more minute.

- Add the onion and mushrooms, salt and fish sauce and stir-fry for about a minute. Remove the vegetable mixture to a bowl and set aside.

- Add another 2/3 tbsp of coconut oil to the wok. When the oil is very hot, add the green pepper and stir-fry for 1 minute.

- Heat a tbsp. of coconut oil, then add the pieces of fish and stir fry until just done and no more. Stir in the cooked veggies until heated through. Enjoy!

SENSATIONAL SALMON

Ingredients:
- 2 salmon filets
- 1 heaping tablespoon coconut flour
- 2 tbsp fresh parsley
- 1 tbsp olive oil
- 1 tbsp mustard powder
- salt and pepper, to taste

Instructions:
- Preheat the oven to 375 F.

- Mix the chopped raw shrimp, egg, onions, parsley, almond meal, 1 tbsp coconut butter, garlic, low sodium salt and pepper. Set aside.

- Lightly season the salmon pieces with salt and pepper. Heat a cast iron pan on high and add the rest of the lard. Pan sear the salmon 1-2 minutes per side.

- Move the salmon to an ovenproof dish and top each piece with 2 tbsp (or more!) of the shrimp topping. Lightly brush the top with a little bit of lard and bake in the oven for 15 minutes.

- Afterwards, set your oven to broil and cook for about 3 more minutes until the top becomes crispy.

CREAMY COCONUT SALMON

Ingredients:
- 1 lb salmon filets
- 1 tsp low sodium salt
- 1 tsp freshly ground black pepper
- 2 tsp olive oil
- 3 cloves fresh garlic (minced)
- 1 large shallot (minced)
- 1 lemon (juice and zest)
- 1 cup unsweetened full-fat coconut milk

Instructions:
- Preheat the oven to 450 degrees.

- Place salmon filets on a parchment or foil lined baking sheet.

- Top your salmon off with olive oil, garlic, and rub into your salmon.

- In a small pan, mix together your coconut milk, lemon, shallot, salt and pepper.

- Bring to a low boil, then remove from heat.

- Pour mixture over salmon. Place in the oven for 10-15 minutes or until salmon is cooked to your preference.

SALMON DILL BONANZA

Ingredients:
- 1 1/2 lbs wild salmon
- zest of one lemon
- 2 tablespoons coconut oil
- 1 tablespoon chopped, fresh dill
- Juice of 1 lemon
- low sodium salt and pepper
- 2 minced garlic cloves

Instructions:
- Preheat the oven to 375°F.

- Place salmon in a shallow baking dish and season with salt and pepper.

- Heat coconut oil in a medium saute pan or skillet over medium heat.

- Add garlic, dill, lemon juice and zest and saute until tender and fragrant, 3-5 minutes.

- Pour mixture over salmon. Bake, uncovered until salmon flakes easily with a fork.

SHRIMP COCKTAIL

Ingredients:

- 1 lb uncooked shrimp, peeled, deveined, and thawed if frozen
- 1 tbsp lemon zest
- salt and pepper to taste
- 1/3 cup olive oil
- 2 tsp dill
- lemon wedges

Instructions:

- Preheat the oven to 400 degrees F. Oil the bottom of a baking dish.

- Rinse the shrimp and pat dry with paper towels. Sprinkle with low salt and pepper and place in the prepared dish.

- Mix together the oil, lemon zest and dill.

- Place about half the mixture on top of the seasoned shrimp.

- Bake for about 10-15 minutes.

- Add the remaining oil/dill/lemon zest mixture on top, and add a squeeze of lemon juice.

GARLICKY SHRIMP

Ingredients:
- 1/2 cup olive oil
- 10 cloves garlic, peeled and thinly sliced
- 1 lb shrimp, peeled, deveined
- salt and pepper to taste
- 1/4 teaspoon paprika

Instructions:
- Preheat the oven to 425 degrees.
- Toss shrimp with oil, garlic, paprika, salt and pepper and spread in a single layer on a rimmed baking sheet.
- Roast, turning once, until shrimp is pink and just cooked through (about 5 or 10 minutes, depending on size of shrimp).

SPICY SCRAMBLED EGGS

Ingredients:
- 1 tablespoon extra virgin olive oil

- 1 red onion, finely chopped
- 1 medium green pepper, cored, seeded, and finely chopped
- 1 chili, seeded and cut into thin strips
- 3 ripe tomatoes, peeled, seeded, and chopped
- Salt and pepper
- 4 large eggs

Instructions:

- Heat the olive oil in a large, heavy, preferably nonstick skillet over medium heat.

- Add the onion and cook until soft, 6 to 7 minutes.

- Add the pepper and chili and continue cooking until soft, another 4 to 5 minutes.

- Add in the tomatoes, and salt and pepper to taste and cook uncovered, over low heat for 10 minutes. Add the eggs, stirring them into the mixture to distribute.

- Cover the skillet and cook until the eggs are set but still fluffy and tender, about 7 to 8 minutes. Serve.

SCRAMBLED EGGS WITH CHILLI

Ingredients:

- 4 fresh green chilies with skins removed
- 2 tbsp coconut oil
- 1 small onion, peeled and finely chopped

- 6 eggs
- 1/4 cup coconut milk
- 1/4 tsp salt

Instructions:

- After removing chili skins, remove and discard seeds and finely chop remaining chili.

- Beat eggs, coconut milk and salt in a bowl and set aside.

- Heat oil in a medium size saucepan over a medium heat.

- Reduce heat to low and add egg mixture to saucepan and mix well.

- Scatter chilies and onion over mixture. Cook over a low heat until eggs are cooked.

- Serve immediately.

BASIL & WALNUT EGGS DIVINE

Ingredients:
- 3 eggs
- 1/2 cup fresh basil, chopped
- 1/3 cup walnuts, chopped
- salt and pepper

Instructions:

- Whisk eggs in a bowl then place in a frying pan on medium heat, stirring constantly.

- When the eggs are almost cooked, add the basil and continue cooking for a further 1 minute or until eggs are fully cooked.

- Add salt and pepper to taste.

- Remove from heat and stir in the walnuts before serving.

INDIAN OMELET

Ingredients:

- 3 Eggs
- 1 Onion, chopped
- 4 Green Chilli (optional)
- 1/4 cup Coconut grated
- Salt, Oil - as required

Instructions:

- Beat the Eggs severely.

- Mix chopped onion, rounded green chili, salt and grated coconuts with eggs.

- Heat oil on a medium-low heat, in a pan.

- Pour the mixture in the form of pancakes and cook it on both sides.

SPICY SPINACH BAKE

Ingredients:

- 6 eggs
- 1 bunch fresh spinach chopped
- 1/2 tsp hot pepper flakes
- Olive oil
- Salt and pepper

Instructions:

- Scramble the eggs in a bowl. Add the spinach, salt and pepper.

- Heat a large non-stick skillet with olive oil.

- When the oil is hot, put the hot pepper flakes in then pour the mixture in. When it starts to cook on the bottom, flip it over.

- Do not overcook, take it out when it is medium scrambled.

- Allow to cool and enjoy.

VEGGIE HASH WITH EGGS

Ingredients:
- 2 tablespoon extra virgin olive oil
- 2 garlic cloves, minced
- 1/4 cup sweet white onion, chopped
- 1 cup yellow squash, chopped
- 1/2 cup mushroom, sliced
- salt and pepper
- 1 cup cherry tomatoes, halved
- 1 cup fresh spinach, chopped
- 4 eggs, poached or cooked any style

Instructions:
- Heat a large non-stick skillet over medium heat. Add olive oil to the pan.

- Add garlic and onion and saute for 2 minutes, then add chopped squash or your favorite vegetable.

- Cook for 2 more minutes, then add mushrooms. Cook for 5 minutes

- At this point add salt and pepper, then add tomatoes and spinach and cook until spinach wilts. Drain well before plating, while finishing this prepare eggs to your liking in another pan.

EGG SALSA

Ingredients:
- 2 lbs fresh ripe tomatoes, peeled and coarsely chopped
- 2 to 3 Serrano or jalapeno chilies, seeded for a milder sauce, and chopped
- 2 garlic cloves, peeled, halved, green shoots removed
- 1/2 small onion, chopped
- 2 tablespoons oil
- salt to taste
- 4 to 8 eggs (to taste)
- Chopped cilantro for garnish

Instructions:
- Place the tomatoes, chilies, garlic and onion in a blender and puree, retaining a bit of texture.

- Heat 1 tablespoon of the oil over high heat in a large, heavy nonstick skillet, until a drop of puree will sizzle when it hits the pan.

- Add the puree and cook, stirring, for four

to ten minutes, until the sauce thickens, darkens and leaves a trough when you run a spoon down the middle of the pan. It should just begin to stick to the pan.

- Season to taste with salt, and remove from the heat. Fry the eggs in a heavy skillet over medium-high heat.

- Use the remaining tablespoon of oil if necessary. Cook them sunny side up, until the whites are solid but the yolks still runny.

- Season with salt and pepper, and turn off the heat. Place one or two fried eggs on each plate. Spoon the hot salsa over the whites of the eggs, leaving the yolks exposed if possible. Sprinkle with cilantro and serve.

MUSHROOMS & EGGS BONANZA

Ingredients:
- 1 medium onion, finely diced
- 1/4 cup coconut oil
- 10-12 medium white mushrooms, finely chopped
- 12 hard boiled eggs, peeled and finely chopped
- Freshly ground black pepper to taste

Instructions:
- Saute the onion in coconut oil until golden brown.

- Add the mushrooms and saute another 5 minutes or so, stirring frequently, until mushrooms are softened and turned dark.

- Remove from heat and let cool. Mix together with the eggs and pepper. Chill until ready to serve.

AVOCADO SHRIMP OMELET

Ingredients:
- 6 eggs
- 2 tbsp chopped parsley
- 2 tbsp lemon juice, divided
- 1/4 tsp salt
- 1/8 tsp cayenne pepper
- 1 large ripe avocado, diced
- 1 1/2 Tbsp. avocado oil

- 3 oz. bay shrimp
- 3 parsley sprigs

Instructions:

- Beat together eggs, parsley, 3/4 of the lemon juice, salt, and cayenne pepper; reserve.

- Gently toss avocado with remaining lemon juice; reserve.

- Heat oil in an omelet pan.

- Pour egg mixture into the pan. Cook over medium heat, lifting edges and tilting pan to allow uncooked egg to run under, until set but still moist on top.

- Scatter reserved avocado and shrimp over omelet.

- Fold omelet in half; heat another minute.

- Slide onto a warmed serving plate; garnish with parsley sprigs.

SPICY TURKEY STIR FRY

Ingredients:
- 2 lbs boneless skinless chicken or turkey breasts, cut into 1-inch slices
- 2 tbsp coconut oil
- 1 tsp cumin seeds
- 1/2 each green, red, and orange bell pepper, thinly sliced
- 1 tsp garam masala
- 2 tsp freshly ground pepper
- low sodium salt, to taste
- Scallions, for garnish

For the marinade:
- 1/2 cup coconut cream
- 1 clove garlic, minced
- 1 tsp ginger, minced
- 1 tbsp freshly ground pepper
- 2 tsp low sodium salt
- 1/4 tsp turmeric

Instructions:
- Place all of the marinade ingredients into a Ziploc bag. Add the chicken, close the bag, and shake to coat.

- Marinate in the refrigerator for at least 30 minutes, or up to 6 hours.

- In a wok or large saute pan, melt the coconut oil over medium-high heat.

- Add the cumin seeds and cook for 2-3 minutes. Add the marinated chicken and let cook for 5 minutes. Stir the chicken until it begins to brown, and then add the peppers, garam masala, and freshly ground pepper.

- Sprinkle with low sodium salt. Cook for 4-5 minutes, stirring regularly, or until the bell pepper is cooked to desired doneness. Serve hot.

TURKEY AND KALE PASTA CASSEROLE

Ingredients:
- 1 lb Turkey breast
- 1 medium spaghetti squash, halved and seeded
- Extra virgin olive oil, for drizzling
- 1 large bunch of kale, de-stemmed, and chopped
- 1/2 red onion, sliced
- 1/3 cup chicken broth
- 1/2 cup coconut milk
- 1 clove garlic, minced
- 2 tsp Italian seasoning
- low sodium salt and freshly ground pepper, to taste

Instructions:
- Preheat the oven to 400 F.

- Using a sharp knife, cut the squash in half lengthwise. Scoop out the seeds and discard. Place the halves, with the cut side up, on a rimmed baking sheet.

- Drizzle with olive oil and sprinkle with low sodium salt and pepper. Roast in the oven for 45-50 minutes.

- Let it cool until you can handle it, then scrape the insides with a fork to shred into strands.

- Melt the coconut oil in a large oven-safe skillet. Add the turkey breast and brown. Once cooked through, transfer to a plate.

- In the same skillet, add the onion and saute for 3 minutes. Next add the garlic, Italian seasoning, and kale and cook for 2-3 minutes.

- Pour in the chicken broth and coconut milk and simmer for 2 minutes. Remove from heat.

- Stir in the cooked turkey. Add the spaghetti squash into the skillet and stir well to combine. Bake for 15-18 minutes.

ROASTED LEMON HERB CHICKEN

Ingredients:
- 12 bone-in chicken thighs and legs
- 1 medium onion, thinly sliced
- 1 tbsp dried rosemary
- 1 tsp dried thyme
- 1 lemon, sliced thin
- 1 orange, sliced thin

For the marinade:
- 5 tbsp extra virgin olive oil
- 6 cloves garlic, minced
- Stevia to taste
- Juice of 1 lemon
- Juice of 1 orange
- 1 tbsp Italian seasoning
- 1 tsp onion powder
- Dash of red pepper flakes

- salt and freshly ground pepper, to taste

Instructions:

- Whisk together all of the marinade ingredients in a small bowl. Place the chicken in a baking dish (or large Ziploc bag) and pour the marinade over it. Marinate for 3 hours overnight.

- Preheat the oven to 400 degrees F. Place the chicken in a baking dish and arrange with the onion, orange, and lemon slices.

- Sprinkle it with thyme, rosemary, salt and pepper. Cover with aluminum foil and bake for 30 minutes.

- Remove the foil, baste the chicken, and bake for another 30 minutes uncovered, until the chicken is cooked through.

BASIL TURKEY WITH ROASTED TOMATOES

Ingredients:
- 2 turkey breasts
- 1 cup mushrooms, chopped
- 1/2 medium onion, chopped
- 1-2 tbsp extra virgin olive oil
- Half cup thinly sliced fresh basil
- salt and pepper, to taste
- 1 pint cherry tomatoes
- Stevia to taste
- Fresh parsley, for garnish

Instructions:

- Preheat the oven to 400 degrees F. Place the tomatoes on a baking sheet and drizzle with olive oil and stevia. Sprinkle with low sodium salt and pepper and toss to coat evenly. Bake for 15-20 minutes until soft.

- While the tomatoes are roasting, heat one tablespoon of olive oil in a large pan over low heat. Add the onions and mushrooms and cook for 10-12 minutes to soften and caramelize, stirring regularly. Clear a space for the chicken.

- Season the turkey with low sodium salt and pepper and then place it in the pan. Simmer for 15 minutes or until the chicken is cooked through. Every 5 minutes or so, spoon the sauce in the pan over the turkey.

- To assemble, divide the tomatoes between two

plates. Place one turkey breast on each and then spoon the onions, mushrooms, and pan drippings over the turkey. Garnish with parsley.

ROASTED STUFFED BELL PEPPERS

Ingredients:
- 5 large bell peppers
- 1 tbsp coconut oil
- 1/2 large onion, diced
- 1 tsp dried oregano
- 1/2 tsp low sodium salt
- 1 lb ground turkey
- 1 large zucchini, halved and diced
- 3 tbsp tomato paste
- Freshly ground black pepper, to taste
- Fresh parsley, for serving

Instructions:

- Preheat the oven to 350 F. Coat a small baking dish with coconut oil spray. Bring a large pot of water to a boil. Cut the stems and top of the peppers off, removing the seeds.

- Place in boiling water for 4-5 minutes. Remove from the water and drain face-down on a paper towel.

- Heat the coconut oil in a large nonstick pan over medium heat. Add in the onion. Saute for 3-4 minutes until the onion begins to soften.

- Stir in the ground turkey, oregano, low sodium salt, and pepper and cook until the turkey is browned.

- Add the zucchini to the skillet as the turkey is finished cooking. Cook everything together until the zucchini is soft, and then drain any juices from the pan.

- Remove the pan from heat and stir in the tomato paste. Bake for 15 minutes.

CHILI-GARLIC VENISON SKEWERS

Ingredients:
- 2 Venison, diced
- 1 tbsp Olive Oil
- 1 tsp Red Chilies, seeds removed & finely chopped
- 4 Garlic Cloves, minced
- 6 tbsp fresh lemon juice

Instructions:
- Preheat the oven to 350 F or preheat the BBQ grill on high heat.

- To make sauce, combine the oil, chilies, garlic, and lemon juice in a small bowl. Set aside for a few minutes.

- Thread diced meat onto skewers and place on an oven tray lined with baking paper.

- Pour chili and garlic sauce over the meat, coating well.

- Bake in the oven for 30-40 minutes. If cooking on a grill, cook meat for 5-6 minutes on each side.

CREAMY CHICKEN CASSEROLE

Ingredients:
- 2 cups cubed cooked chicken
- 1 1/2 cups cooked butternut squash
- 1/2 cup coconut cream
- 1/4 cup coconut oil, melted
- 1 heaping cup green peas, fresh or frozen
- 1 tbsp apple cider vinegar
- 1/2 tsp low sodium salt
- 1/2 tsp oregano
- 1/2 tsp thyme
- 1 tbsp fresh parsley

Instructions:
- In a large bowl, mash the butternut squash. Stir in the coconut cream, oil, vinegar, low sodium salt, oregano, and thyme.

- Once everything is combined, add in chicken and peas.

- Place the mixture into a large saucepan and cook over medium heat for 5- 8 minutes.

- Top with fresh parsley and serve warm.

SPAGHETTI WITH TURKEY BALLS

Ingredients:
- 1 spaghetti squash
- Extra virgin olive oil,
- salt and pepper
- 1 tsp dried or fresh oregano

For the sauce:
- 1 lb ground turkey
- 1 small onion, chopped
- 4 cloves garlic, minced
- 1 tbsp coconut oil
- 1 tomato, chopped
- 1/2 jar of tomato sauce
- 1 tbsp Italian seasoning
- low sodium salt and pepper to taste
- Fresh basil

Instructions:

- Preheat the oven to 400 F. Using a sharp knife, cut the squash in half lengthwise. Scoop out the seeds and discard. Place the halves with the cut side up on a rimmed baking sheet. Drizzle with olive oil and season with salt, pepper, and oregano. Roast the squash in the oven for 40-45 minutes, until you can poke the squash easily with a fork.

- Let it cool until you can handle it safely. Then scrape the insides with a fork to shred the squash into strands. While the spaghetti squash is roasting, melt coconut oil in a large skillet over medium heat.

- Add chopped onion and garlic and cook for 4-5 minutes. Add ground turkey and brown the meat, stirring occasionally. Season with low sodium salt and pepper.

- Add the chopped tomato, tomato sauce, and Italian seasoning and stir to combine. Simmer on low heat, stirring occasionally, while the spaghetti squash finishes roasting. Serve over spaghetti squash.

ZUCCHINI PASTA AND TURKEY BOLOGNESE

Ingredients:
- 4 medium zucchini

For the sauce:
- 1 lb ground turkey
- 1 small onion, chopped
- 4 cloves garlic, minced
- 1 tbsp coconut oil
- 1 tomato, chopped
- 1/2 jar of tomato sauce
- 1 tbsp Italian seasoning
- salt and pepper to taste
- Fresh basil, for garnish

Instructions:
- Use a julienne peeler to slice the zucchini into noodles, stopping when you reach the seeds. Set aside.

- Add zucchini noodles to a skillet and saute over medium heat for 4-5 minutes.

- Melt coconut oil in a large skillet over medium heat. Add chopped onion and garlic and cook for 4-5 minutes.

- Add ground turkey and brown the meat, stirring occasionally. Season with salt and pepper.

- Add the chopped tomato, tomato sauce, and Italian seasoning and stir to combine. Simmer on low heat, stirring occasionally.

- Add the sauce to the zoodles and enjoy!

TURKEY STIR-FRY

Ingredients:
- 2 tbsp. of coconut oil
- 2 cloves of garlic (thinly sliced)
- 1 inch ginger (finely grated)
- 2-3 green (spring) onions (sliced into long slivers)
- 1 carrot (coarsely grated)
- 1 green pepper (sliced into thin, long pieces)
- 1 turkey breast (cut into bite-sized pieces)
- 1/4 cup water
- 2 tbsp veggie broth
- A few drops of toasted sesame oil

Instructions:

- Heat 2 tbsp coconut oil in a wok or large pan. Add the sliced garlic and grated ginger to the wok and stir-fry for 30 seconds.

- Add the green onion and stir-fry 1 more minute.

- Add the carrot and stir-fry for about one minute. You want it just barely cooked, not limp and soggy. Remove the vegetable mixture to a bowl and set aside.

- Add another 2/3 tbsp. of coconut oil to the wok. When the oil is very hot, add the green pepper and stir-fry for 1 minute.

- Heat a tbsp. of coconut oil, then add the pieces of turkey breast and stir fry.

- Add the sesame oil, and serve.

CREAMY CURRY STIR FRY

Ingredients:
- 2 cooked chicken breasts
- 3 carrots, chopped
- 3 sticks celery, chopped
- 1-2 heads broccoli, chopped
- 1/2 medium onion, chopped
- 2 cloves garlic
- 1/2 cup coconut milk
- 2 tbsp turmeric
- 2 tbsp curry powder
- 2 tbsp coconut oil

Instructions:
- Put coconut oil in a pan and add chopped onion. Cook until onion softens up, add garlic and cook for an additional few minutes.

- Next up, add in the carrots, celery, and broccoli. Cook until they have softened a bit (but are not fully cooked).

- Shred the cooked chicken up into small pieces for the stir fry and add the coconut milk, other milk, and curry spices.

- Stir everything thoroughly, simmer for 5-10 minutes or until everything is cooked to your liking, and serve hot.

- Add cauliflower rice (grated cauliflower boiled for 3 minutes)

TURKEY SCRAMBLE

Ingredients:
- 1 lb ground turkey
- 2 medium yellow onions
- 2 bell peppers
- 2 medium squash or zucchini
- 1 large hand-full of fresh spinach
- 1 tablespoon each of: (cumin, chili powder, garlic powder)
- Salt to taste
- cilantro

Instructions:
- Brown the turkey until well cooked in a large skillet or wok over medium high heat.

- Remove and add thinly sliced onions, peppers, squash/zucchini to the pan and saute, stirring constantly, until starting to soften.

- Return the turkey to the pan and add fresh

spinach. Season to taste and continue to cook until spinach is wilted.

- Remove and serve with any desired toppings.

CHICKEN SALAD

Ingredients:
- olive oil spray
- 2 tsp olive oil
- 16 oz skinless boneless chicken breasts, cut into chunks
- salt and pepper to taste
- 4 cups shredded romaine
- 1 cup shredded red cabbage

For the Skinny Sauce:
- 2 1/2 tbsp paleo mayonnaise
- 2 tbsp scallions, chopped fine plus more for topping
- 1 1/2 tsp chili flakes

Instructions:
- Preheat the oven to 425°F. Spray a baking sheet with olive oil spray.

- Season chicken with low sodium salt and pepper, olive oil and mix well so the olive oil evenly coats all of the chicken.

- Meanwhile combine the sauce in a medium bowl. When the chicken is ready, drizzle it over the top and enjoy!

MELTING MUSTARD CHICKEN

Ingredients:
- 8 small chicken thighs, skin removed
- 3 tsp mustard powder
- 1 tbsp paleo mayonnaise
- 1 clove garlic, crushed
- Juice and zest of 1 lime
- 3/4 tsp pepper
- Salt
- dried parsley

Instructions:
- Preheat the oven to 400°. Rinse the chicken and remove the skin and all fat.
- Pat dry and place in a large bowl and season generously with low sodium salt. In a small bowl combine mustard, mayonnaise, lime juice, lime zest, garlic and pepper. Mix well. Pour over chicken, tossing well to coat.
- Spray a large baking pan with a little Pam to prevent sticking since all the fat and skin was removed from the chicken. Place chicken to fit in a single layer.
- Top the chicken with dried parsley. Bake until cooked through, about 30- 35 minutes.
- Finish the chicken under the broiler until it is golden brown. Serve chicken with the pan juices drizzled over the top.

TURKEY WITH ROASTED VEGETABLES

Ingredients:
- 1 lb Turkey Breasts
- 20 medium asparagus, ends trimmed, cut in half
- 3 red bell peppers
- 1 cup carrots, sliced in half long way
- 2 red onions, chopped in large chunks
- 10 oz sliced mushrooms
- 1/2 cup plus 2 tbsp rice vinegar
- 1/4 cup extra virgin olive oil
- 1 tsp stevia
- salt and pepper
- 3 tbsp fresh rosemary
- 2 cloves garlic, smashed and sliced
- 2 tbsp oregano or thyme
- 4 leaves fresh sage, chopped

Instructions:
- Preheat the oven to 425°. Wash and dry the chicken well with a paper towel. Combine all the ingredients together and using your hands and arrange in a large roasting pan.

- The vegetables should not touch the turkey or it will steam instead of roast.

- All ingredients should be spread out in a single layer. If necessary use two baking sheets or disposable tins to achieve this. Bake for 35 - 40 minutes.

GRILLED OSTRICH STEAK

Ingredients:
- 6 medium ostrich steaks
- 1 tbsp vinegar
- garlic powder
- black pepper ground to taste
- oregano
- 2 tbsp olive oil

Instructions:
- Season ostrich with vinegar and olive oil.

- Add garlic powder, oregano and mix well, marinate for at least 20 minutes.

- Broil or grill on low until the ostrich is cooked through, careful not to burn. Enjoy with green salad.

LEMONY CHICKEN AND ASPARAGUS

Ingredients:
- 1 1/2 lbs skinless chicken breast, cut into 1-inch cubes
- salt to taste
- 1/2 cup reduced-sodium chicken broth
- 2 tbsp reduced-sodium soy sauce (or Tamari sauce)

- 2 tbsp water
- 1 tbsp olive oil, divided
- 1 bunch asparagus, ends trimmed, cut into 2-inch pieces
- 6 cloves garlic, chopped
- 1 tbsp fresh ginger
- 3 tbsp fresh lemon juice
- fresh black pepper, to taste

Instructions:

- Lightly season the chicken with low sodium salt. In a small bowl, combine chicken broth and soy sauce. In a second small bowl combine the cornstarch and water and mix well to combine.

- Heat a large non-stick wok over medium-high heat, when hot add 1 teaspoon of the oil, then add the asparagus and cook until tender-crisp, about 3 to 4 minutes. Add the garlic and ginger and cook until golden, about 1 minute. Set aside.

- Increase the heat to high, then add 1 teaspoon of oil and half of the chicken and cook until browned and cooked through, about 4 minutes on each side. Remove and set aside and repeat with the remaining oil and chicken. Set aside.

- Add the soy sauce mixture; bring to a boil and cook for about 1-1/2 minutes. Add lemon juice and stir well, when it simmers return the chicken and asparagus to the wok and mix well, remove from heat and serve.

CHICKEN SOUP

Ingredients:
- 5 cups reduced sodium chicken broth
- 2 cups shredded chicken breast
- 1 tomato, diced
- 2 cloves garlic, minced
- 1-1/2 cups scallions, chopped fine
- 1/3 cup cilantro, chopped fine
- 4 lime wedges
- 2 tsp olive oil
- salt and pepper to taste
- pinch cumin

Instructions:
- In a large pot, heat oil over medium heat. Add 1 cup of scallions and garlic.

- Saute about 2 minutes then add tomatoes and saute another minute, until soft. Add chicken stock, cumin and chili powder and bring to a boil.

- Simmer, covered on low for about 15-20 minutes.

- Ladle 1 cup chicken broth over the chicken and serve with a lime wedge.

PAPRIKA CHICKEN

Ingredients:
- 3 boneless skinless chicken thighs, all fat trimmed
- 8 cups water
- 1 tbsp low salt chicken broth
- 1 small onion
- 2 scallions
- 1/4 cup chopped cilantro
- 3 cloves garlic
- 1 medium ripe tomato
- 1 tsp garlic powder
- 1 tsp cumin
- 1/4 tsp oregano
- 1 tsp ground Spanish paprika
- salt to taste

Instructions:
- In a large pot combine paprika, chicken, water and chicken broth.

- Bring to a boil, covered over medium-low heat until chicken is cooked, about 20 minutes. Remove the chicken and shred, return to the pot.

- Meanwhile, in a chopper or by hand, mince the onions, scallions, cilantro, garlic, and tomato.

- Add garlic powder, cumin, oregano and cook, covered for 25 more minutes, adding more water as needed if too thick.

CHICKEN VEGGIES SOUP

Ingredients:
- 1 teaspoon olive oil
- 1 cup chopped carrots
- 1 cup chopped onions
- 1/2 cup chopped celery
- 2 chopped cloves garlic
- 1-1/2 lbs skinless bone-in chicken breast
- 7 cups reduced sodium chicken broth
- 1/4 cup chopped parsley
- 2 bay leaves
- fresh ground black pepper, to taste

Instructions:

- Heat a large heavy pot on medium heat. Add the oil, carrots, onion, celery and garlic to the pot and stir.

- Add chicken, broth, parsley, and bay leaves and bring to a boil. When boiling, reduce heat to low and cover.

- Simmer over low heat until the chicken and vegetables are tender, about 30 minutes.

- Remove the chicken, shred or cut the meat, discard the bones and return the chicken to the pot, adjust the salt if needed and add fresh ground pepper.

- Simmer for 20 minutes . Discard the bay leaves and serve.

OYSTER CHICKEN

Ingredients:
- 6 chicken thighs, skin and fat removed
- olive oil spray
- 1 red bell pepper, chopped
- 1 cup chopped oyster mushrooms
- 1/2 onion, chopped
- 2 garlic cloves, finely chopped
- 28 oz canned crushed tomatoes
- 1/4 cup fat free chicken broth, more if needed
- 1 tsp dried oregano leaves
- 1/4 cup fresh chopped basil leaves
- salt and freshly ground black pepper to taste

Instructions:
- Season chicken with low sodium salt and pepper. In a large heavy saute pan, heat the pan over a medium-high flame and spray with cooking oil.
- Add the chicken pieces to the pan and saute just until brown, about 3-4 minutes per side.

- Add the peppers, onion and garlic to the pan and saute over medium heat until the onion is tender, about 3-4 minutes, then add mushrooms and cook for another 2-3 minutes.

- Season with low sodium salt and pepper. Add the tomatoes, broth, and oregano.

- Cover the pan and bring the sauce to a simmer. Continue simmering over low heat until the chicken is just cooked through, about 25 minutes. Add the chopped basil 5 minutes before the sauce is done.

CHICKEN COCONUT DIVINE

Ingredients:
- 1 tbsp olive oil
- 1/2 tsp roasted cumin
- 1-1/2 tsp garam masala
- 2 tsp curry powder
- 1/2 onion, minced
- 5 cloves garlic, minced
- 1 large tomato, chopped
- 2 tbsp fresh cilantro, chopped
- 1/2 cup light coconut milk
- 3/4 cup water
- 6 skinless chicken thighs
- salt to taste

Instructions:
- Add oil to a large pan, on medium heat. When oil is hot add onion and garlic and saute. Add cumin, masala and curry powder and mix well.

- Place chicken in the pan and season with low sodium salt. Mix together with all spices and brown on both sides for a few minutes.

- Add tomatoes, cilantro, water, coconut milk and adjust low sodium salt to taste. Mix all ingredients and cover pan, simmer on low until chicken is cooked through, about 20 minutes.

- Serve with Cauliflower rice if desired

TURKEY LETTUCE FAJITAS

Ingredients:
- 16 oz turkey breasts
- 1 red bell pepper, cut into strips
- 1 green pepper, cut into strips
- 1 medium onion, cut into strips
- 3 tbsp lime juice
- 1 tsp ground cumin
- 1 tsp garlic powder
- A Pinch of chili powder
- salt and pepper to taste
- 2 tsp olive oil
- 8 lettuce leaves

Instructions:

- Marinate the turkey with lime juice, and season with chili powder, low sodium salt, pepper, garlic powder and cumin.

- Season vegetables with salt and pepper and toss with olive oil.

- Cook onions and peppers outside in a large skillet over medium heat for 16 to 18 minutes, covered until they are soft.

- Grill turkey meat until cooked through, about 10 minutes on each side.

- Transfer to a cutting board when done and

cut into strips. Once cooked, combine with the peppers and onions. Serve immediately inside lettuce cups.

CHICKEN JEREZ

Ingredients:
- 4 large chicken breast halves, thinly sliced in 3
- 3 tbsp lemon juice
- 1/2 lemon sliced thin
- 1/3 cup Jerez Sherry
- 15 oz low sodium chicken broth
- l salt and fresh pepper to taste
- 3 tbsp fresh chopped parsley
- 1 tbsp olive oil

Instructions:

- Season the chicken with low sodium salt and pepper. Heat a very large non-stick pan over medium heat. When hot spray with cooking spray to lightly coat the bottom of the pan.

- Saute chicken 2-3 minutes on each side. When cooked, transfer onto a plate. Spray the pan again and repeat until all chicken has been cooked.

- Once all chicken is cooked, place the chicken broth in the bowl and to the pan along with the juice of the lemon, sherry, lemon slices, parsley and butter and simmer over medium heat for about 2 minutes so it reduces slightly.

- Turn off heat. Return chicken to the pan to combine with the sauce.

LEEKY CHICKEN

Ingredients:
- 1 or 2 leeks white part and light green only
- 6 skinless chicken breast cutlets, sliced thin
- 2 tsp olive oil, divided
- 1 clove garlic, minced
- 2 oz sun dried tomatoes (not in oil), sliced
- 1/4 cup white wine
- 1/2 cup fat free low sodium chicken broth
- salt and pepper to taste
- 2 tbsp chopped fresh parsley

Instructions:

- Cut off green tops of leek and remove outer tough leaves. Cut off root and cut leeks in half lengthwise. Fan out the leeks and rinse well under running water, leaving them intact. Slice leeks into 1/4-inch slices. Set aside.

- Preheat the oven to 200°F. Season chicken with low sodium salt and pepper. Heat a large skillet on medium heat; when hot add 1 tsp olive oil. Add chicken to the skillet and cook on medium heat for about 3 - 4 minutes on each side, or until chicken is no longer pink. Set aside in a warm oven.

- Add additional oil to the skillet, then garlic and cook for a few seconds; add leeks, low sodium salt and pepper. Saute stirring occasionally until golden, about 5 minutes.

- Add sun dried tomatoes, wine, chicken broth, parsley; stir the pan with a wooden spoon, breaking up any brown bits from the bottom of the pan. Cook for 2 more minutes or until the liquid reduces almost by half. Top the chicken with the sun dried tomatoes/leeks mixture and serve with a green salad.

ZESTY CHICKEN LEMON

Ingredients:
- 2 skinless chicken breasts, all fat trimmed
- freshly ground black pepper
- 2 egg whites
- 3 tbsp olive oil
- juice of 2 lemons, lemon halves reserved
- 1/4 cup dry white wine
- 1/2 cup reduced sodium chicken broth
- 1 tbsp capers
- Sliced lemon, for serving
- Chopped fresh parsley leaves, for serving

Instructions:
- Cut chicken into 4 cutlets, then place cutlets between 2 sheets of parchment paper or plastic wrap and pound out to 1/4-inch thick. Sprinkle both sides with low sodium salt and pepper.

- Heat a large saute pan over medium to medium-low heat. Spray a generous amount of olive oil spray on one side of the chicken, and lay it in the pan, oil side down. Spray the top of the chicken generously to coat and cook for 2-3 minutes on each side, until cooked through. Set aside until you make the sauce.

- For the sauce, clean the saute pan. Over medium heat, add olive oil, add the lemon juice, wine, chicken broth and the reserved lemon halves, low sodium salt, and pepper.

- Boil over high heat until reduced in half, about 2 minutes. Discard the lemon halves, add the capers and serve one chicken cutlet on each plate. Spoon on the sauce and serve with a slice of lemon and a sprinkling of fresh parsley.

CHICKY SOUP

Ingredients:
- 2 chicken breasts, on the bone, skin removed
- 1 tsp seasoning low sodium salt
- 1/2 tsp olive oil
- 1 large onion, chopped
- 2 celery stalks, chopped
- 3 garlic cloves, chopped
- 1/2 tsp dried oregano
- 1/2 tsp dried thyme
- 1/2 tsp ground cumin
- 6 cups reduced sodium chicken broth
- 1 large sweet potato, peeled and diced
- 3 cups kale, roughly chopped
- 1 fresh jalapeno, sliced in half lengthwise
- 1/4 cup fresh cilantro

Instructions:

- Season the chicken with the salt and set aside while you prep all your vegetables.

- Heat a large nonstick pot over medium-low heat, add the oil and the onions and celery and cook until soft and golden, about 8 to 10 minutes, then add the garlic and dry spices and cook for 2 to 3 minutes.

- Add the chicken broth, chicken, jalapeno and cilantro. Cover and cook for 20 minutes, then add the sweet potato and kale and cook until the sweet potatoes are tender and the chicken is cooked, about 25 to 30 minutes.

- Remove the chicken, shred or cut up and discard the bones. Return to the pot, discard the jalapeno and serve the soup into 6 bowls.

CHICKEN ZOODLES

Ingredients:

For the sauce:
- 1/2 cup reduced sodium chicken broth
- 1 tbsp reduced sodium soy sauce
- 1/2 tbsp rice wine

For the zoodles:
- 2 medium zucchini, ends trimmed
- 8 oz skinless, boneless chicken breast, cut into thin short strips
- salt, to taste
- 2 tsp olive oil, divided
- 3/4 cup sliced bok choy
- 1/2 cup sliced mushrooms such as shiitake
- 1/2 cup shredded carrots
- 3 scallions, sliced into 1-inch pieces on the diagonal
- 1/2 tbsp grated fresh ginger
- 2 garlic cloves, chopped
- 1 tbsp almond flour

Instructions:
- For the sauce - in a medium bowl, combine the

chicken broth, soy sauce and 2 tablespoons of water. Use 1 tablespoon almond flour to thicken Using a spiralizer fitted with a shredder blade, or a mandolin fitted with a julienne blade, cut the zucchini into long spaghetti-like strips.

- Season chicken with salt. Heat a large nonstick wok over high heat. Add 1 tsp of the oil and the chicken. Cook until browned on both sides and opaque throughout, 2 to 3 minutes. Set aside.

- Add the remaining oil, bok choy, mushroom, carrots, scallions, ginger and garlic. Cook until crisp tender, 2 to 3 minutes. Set aside with the chicken. Pour the sauce mixture into the wok and cook, stirring, until thickened and bubbling, 1 to 1- 1/2 minutes.

- Add the zucchini noodles to the sauce, mixing so the zucchini is covered in sauce, and cook until the zucchini is tender, 2 minutes.

- Add the chicken and vegetables to combine, then divide between two serving bowls.

COCONUT TURKEY SALAD

Ingredients:
- 6 turkey breasts
- 6 tbsp shredded coconut
- Pinch of salt
- olive oil spray

- 6 cups mixed baby greens
- 3/4 cup shredded carrots
- 1 large tomato, sliced
- 1 small cucumber, sliced
- 2 beaten egg whites

For the Vinaigrette:
- 1 tbsp oil
- Stevia to taste
- 1 tbsp white vinegar
- 2 tsp mustard powder

Instructions:

- Whisk all vinaigrette ingredients; set aside. Preheat oven to 375°F.

- Combine coconut flakes and salt in a bowl. Put egg whites in another bowl.

- Lightly season chicken with salt. Dip the chicken in the egg, then in the coconut flake mixture. Place chicken on a cookie sheet lined with parchment for easy cleanup. Lightly spray with olive oil spray and bake for 30 minutes turning halfway, or until chicken is cooked through.

- Place 2 cups of baby greens on each plate. Divide carrots, cucumber, and tomato evenly between each plate. When chicken is ready, slice on the diagonal and place on top of greens. Heat dressing and divide equally between each salad; a little over 1 tbsp each.

CREAMY CHICKEN MUSHROOM SOUP

Ingredients:
- 4 cups water
- 1 celery stalk, cut in half
- 5 oz shiitake mushrooms, sliced
- 4 tsp Chicken Bouillon (low salt)
- 7 oz skinless chicken breast
- 1 tbsp fresh parsley, chopped
- 1 tbsp almond flour

Instructions:

- Place cold water and flour in a blender and blend until smooth; pour into a medium pot and set heat to medium.

- Add celery, mushrooms, chicken bouillon and bring to a boil. Add chicken, cover and simmer on low 15 minutes, or until chicken is cooked through.

- Remove chicken and set aside; continue to cook the remaining soup an additional 5 minutes, until vegetables are soft.

- Place celery and 1 cup of soup into the blender; blend until smooth, then return to the pot and simmer for a few minutes.

- Shred or cut the chicken into small pieces and

add back to the soup, garnish with fresh parsley.

FILIPINO STYLE CHICKEN

Ingredients:
- 8 chicken legs on the bone (skin removed)
- 1/3 cup low sodium soy sauce
- 1/3 cup apple cider vinegar
- 1 small head of garlic, crushed
- 6 ground peppercorns
- 4 bay leaves
- 1 jalapeno, chopped (optional)

Instructions:

- Marinate chicken in vinegar, soy sauce, garlic, jalapeno and pepper, for at least one hour (overnight is ideal).

- Add chicken, 1/2 cup water, bay leaves and marinade into a deep nonstick skillet and cook on medium-low heat. Cover and cook until the meat is tender, about 45 minutes.

- Remove the cover and cook for an additional 15 minutes, until the sauce reduces. Discard bay leaves and serve over cauliflower rice.

CHINESE CHICKEN LEGS

Ingredients:
- 3 lbs chicken legs (thighs and legs attached), fat trimmed

For the marinade:
- 6 cloves of garlic
- 1 large shallot
- 1 tbsp grated fresh ginger
- Stevia to taste
- 1/4 cup reduced sodium soy sauce
- 1/2 tsp Chinese five-spice powder
- freshly ground black pepper

Instructions:
- In a blender combine the marinade ingredients; blend until smooth.
- Place the chicken in a large, resealable zip-top bag or container and pour in the marinade. Toss the chicken inside the bag to cover evenly with the marinade and refrigerate for 6-8 hours or as long as overnight.
- Preheat the oven to 400°F. Place the chicken on a rack in a foil lined roasting pan. Create a loose tent over the chicken with foil.
- Roast the chicken in the center of the oven for 30 minutes; remove foil and continue to cook, basting occasionally until the internal temperature is 165°- 170°F, about 45 minutes longer (Insert thermometer between the leg and the thigh).

JAMAICAN CHICKEN

ingredients:
- 6 bone-in chicken legs with thighs attached, skin removed
- 1 lime or 1/4 cup lime juice
- 1 large tomato, chopped
- 4 medium scallions, chopped
- 1 large onion, chopped
- 2 garlic cloves, chopped
- 1/2 - 1 hot chili, chopped
- 4 sprigs fresh thyme or 2 tsp dried thyme
- 2 tbsp low sodium soy sauce
- 1 tsp coconut oil 1 medium carrot, chopped finely
- 2 tsp almond flour
- 1 1/2 cups unsweetened light coconut milk
- 1/4 tsp low sodium salt

Instructions:
- Squeeze lime over chicken and rub well. Drain off excess lime juice.
- Combine tomato, scallion, onion, garlic, chili pepper, thyme and soy sauce in a large bowl and add to the chicken. Cover and marinate for at least one hour.

- Heat oil in a large saucepan. Shake off the seasonings as you remove each piece of chicken from the marinade, reserving the marinade for later.

- Lightly brown the chicken on medium-high heat. When browned on all sides, pour the marinade over the chicken and add the carrots. Stir and cook over medium heat for 10 minutes.

- Mix flour and coconut milk and add to stew, stirring constantly. Reduce heat to low and cook for an additional 20 minutes or until tender, add salt to taste.

CITRUS CHICKEN

Ingredients:

For the lemon Sauce:
- 1/3 cup freshly squeezed lemon juice
- 1/4 cup reduced sodium chicken broth
- 2 tbsp soy or Tamari sauce
- Stevia to taste
- 1 tbsp Chinese rice wine
- Chili flakes to taste
- 1 tbsp rice vinegar
- 1/4 tsp white pepper

For the chicken:
- 20 oz skinless, boneless chicken breast, cut into small cubes
- salt, to taste
- 1 tbsp sesame oil
- 4 cloves minced garlic

- 1-inch grated ginger
- 1 tsp grated lemon zest
- 2 tbsp chopped scallions
- 1/2 tsp sesame seeds, for garnish

Instructions:

- Mix the lemon sauce ingredients and set aside. Season the chicken lightly with salt and coat evenly with corn starch, set aside.
- Heat 1 tsp of sesame oil and add half of the chicken. Cook 2 to 3 minutes on each side until well browned, set aside. Add 1 tsp of oil and chicken and repeat cooking 2 to 3 minutes on each side. Set aside with the rest of the chicken.
- Add remaining oil and stir-fry the minced garlic and ginger until fragrant. Add the lemon zest then return the chicken to the pan.
- Stir the chicken then add the sauce and cook until the sauce thickens.
- Serve and garnish with the scallion and sesame seeds.

CHICKEN PINEAPPLE

Ingredients:
- 1 lb boneless skinless chicken breast, cut into 1-inch cubes
- 1 tbsp oil, divided
- 1 tsp minced garlic
- 1 tsp minced ginger
- 2 cups cubed assorted colors bell peppers
- 1 chopped red chili pepper
- 1 cup fresh pineapple chunks
- 1/2 tsp chili flakes (optional)
- cilantro leaves (for garnish)

Instructions:
- Heat 1/2 tablespoon of the oil in a large nonstick skillet on medium-high heat. Add garlic and ginger; stir fry for 30 seconds.

- Add bell peppers, chili pepper if using and pineapple; stir fry 3 to 5 minutes or until peppers are tender-crisp. Add sauce; cook and stir until heated through. Remove from the skillet.

- Heat remaining oil in the skillet. Add chicken; stir fry 5 minutes or until cooked through. Return bell pepper mixture to skillet; stir fry until well blended. Garnish with cilantro.

CHICKEN PEANUT LETTUCE WRAPS

Ingredients:

For the Peanut Sauce:
- 1/2 cup reduced-sodium chicken broth
- 1 tbsp peanut butter
- Stevia to taste
- 1 tbsp soy sauce
- 1/2 tbsp freshly grated ginger
- 1 crushed clove garlic

For the Chicken
- 16 oz ground chicken
- 4 cloves garlic, crushed
- 1 tbsp fresh ginger, grated
- 1 tbsp soy sauce
- 3/4 cups shredded carrots
- 2/3 cup scallions, chopped
- 3/4 cup shredded red cabbage
- 2 tbsp chopped peanuts

- cilantro leaves, for garnish
- 4 lime wedges
- 8 iceberg lettuces outer leaves

Instructions:

- Make the peanut sauce; in a small saucepan combine chicken broth, stevia, 1 tablespoon soy sauce, 1/2 tablespoon fresh ginger, and 1 clove crushed garlic and simmer over medium-low heat stirring occasionally until sauce becomes smooth and thickens, about 6 to 8 minutes.

- Meanwhile, heat a large non-stick skillet or wok over high medium until hot. When hot, spray with oil and saute the chicken until cooked through and browned, breaking it up as it cooks; add the remaining garlic and ginger and saute 1 minute. Add the soy sauce, cook for 1 minute.

- Add the shredded carrots, and 1/2 cup of the scallions and saute until tender crisp, about 1-2 minutes. Set aside.

- Divide the chicken equally between 8 lettuce leaves, top each with shredded cabbage, remaining scallions, drizzle with peanut sauce, chopped peanuts and cilantro, for garnish and serve with lime wedges.

THAI BAKED FISH WITH SQUASH NOODLES

Ingredients:

- 1 medium spaghetti squash
- Extra virgin olive oil, for drizzling

- salt and pepper to taste
- 1 tbsp coconut oil
- 1/2 large onion, finely chopped
- 1 head broccoli, cut into florets
- 2 heads baby bok choy, sliced into 1-inch strips
- 4 scallions, sliced
- 1/4 tsp red pepper flakes
- 1/3 cup cashews, toasted and chopped

For the Sauce:
- 1 tsp lime juice
- 1/2-inch piece minced fresh ginger
- 1 clove garlic, minced
- 1/2 tsp red wine vinegar
- 3 tbsp almond butter
- 3 tbsp coconut milk

For the Fish:
- 2 fish filets

Instructions:

- Preheat the oven to 400 degrees F. Place squash in the microwave for 3- 4 minutes to soften. Using a sharp knife, cut the squash in half lengthwise.

- Scoop out the seeds and discard. Place the halves, with the cut side up, on a rimmed baking sheet. Drizzle with olive oil and sprinkle with low sodium salt and pepper.

- Roast in the oven for 45-50 minutes, until

you can poke the squash easily with a fork. Let cool until you can handle it safely. Then scrape the insides with a fork to shred the squash into strands.

- Combine the lime juice, ginger, garlic, and red wine vinegar in a blender or food processor until smooth. Add the almond butter and coconut milk and blend until completely combined.

- Melt the coconut oil in a large pan over medium heat. Add the onion and cook for 5-6 minutes until translucent. Add the broccoli and saute for 8-10 minutes, until just tender. Then stir in the bok choy and cook for 3-4 minutes until wilted. Lastly add the cooked spaghetti squash into the pan and stir to combine.
- Top the spaghetti squash mixture with the scallions and cilantro. Sprinkle with roasted cashews and drizzle with Thai sauce.

- Place the whole fish under the grill at 200 F for 25 minutes topped with 1 tbsp of olive oil, fresh pressed garlic and cayenne pepper.

MEXICAN STYLE PRAWN

Ingredients:
- 1 tbsp extra virgin olive oil
- 1 tsp chili powder
- 1 tsp low sodium salt
- 1 lb medium shrimp, peeled and deveined

- 1 avocado, pitted and diced
- Shredded lettuce, for serving
- Fresh cilantro, for serving
- 1 lime, cut into wedges

For the tortillas:
- 6 egg whites
- 1/4 cup coconut flour
- 1/4 cup almond milk
- 1/2 tsp low sodium salt
- 1/2 tsp cumin
- 1/4 tsp chili powder

Instructions:

- Combine all of the tortilla ingredients together in a small bowl and mix well. Allow the batter to sit for approximately 10 minutes to allow the flour to soak up some of the moisture, and then stir again. The consistency should be similar to crepe batter.

- While the batter is resting, heat a skillet to medium-high. Mix together the olive oil, chili powder, and low sodium salt and toss with the shrimp to coat. Cook in the skillet for 1-2 minutes per side, until translucent. Set aside.

- Coat the pan with coconut oil spray. Pour about 1/4 cup of batter onto the skillet, turning the pan with your wrist to help it spread out in a thin, even layer.

- Cook for 1-2 minutes, loosening the sides with a spatula. When the bottom has firmed up, carefully flip over and cook for another 2-3 minutes until lightly browned, then set aside on a plate. Repeat with remaining batter.

- Top each tortilla with cooked shrimp, shredded lettuce, avocado, and cilantro. Serve with a lime wedge.

SALMON WITH LEMON AND THYME

Ingredients:
- 32 oz salmon
- 1 lemon, sliced thin
- 1 tbsp capers
- salt and freshly ground pepper
- 1 tbsp fresh thyme
- Olive oil

Instructions:
- Line a rimmed baking sheet with parchment paper and place salmon, skin side down, on the prepared baking sheet.

- Season salmon with low sodium salt and pepper. Arrange capers on the salmon, and top with sliced lemon and thyme.

- Place the baking sheet in a cold oven, then turn heat to 400 F. Bake for 25 minutes. Serve immediately.

SHRIMP SCAMPI IN SPAGHETTI SAUCE

Ingredients:

For the Spaghetti:
- 1 spaghetti squash
- Extra virgin olive oil, for drizzling
- salt and pepper
- 1 tsp dried oregano
- 1 tsp dried basil

For the shrimp scampi:
- 8 oz. shrimp, peeled and deveined
- 3 tbsp butter
- 1 tbsp extra virgin olive oil
- 2 cloves garlic, minced
- Pinch of red pepper flakes
- salt and pepper, to taste
- 1 tbsp fresh parsley, chopped
- Juice of 1 lemon
- Zest of half a lemon

Instructions:

- Preheat the oven to 400 F. Place squash in the microwave for 3- 4 minutes to soften. Using a sharp knife, cut the squash in half lengthwise. Scoop out the seeds and discard. Place the halves, with the cut side up, on a rimmed baking sheet.

- Drizzle with olive oil and sprinkle with seasonings. Roast in the oven for 45- 50 minutes, until you can poke the squash easily with a fork.

- Let it cool until you can handle it safely. Then scrape the insides with a fork to shred the squash into strands.

- After removing spaghetti squash from the oven, melt the butter and olive oil in a skillet over medium heat.

- Add in the garlic and saute for 2-3 minutes. Then add in the shrimp, low sodium salt, pepper, and a pinch of red pepper flakes.

- Cook for 5 minutes, until the shrimp is cooked through. Remove from heat and add in the desired amount of cooked spaghetti squash. Toss with lemon juice and zest. Top with parsley.

SHRIMP SCAMPI

Ingredients:
- 4 tsp olive oil
- 1 1/4 lbs med raw shrimp, peeled and deveined
- 6-8 garlic cloves, minced
- 1/2 cup low sodium chicken broth
- 1/4 cup fresh lemon juice
- 1/4 cup + 1 tbsp minced parsley
- 1/4 tsp low sodium salt
- 1/4 tsp freshly ground pepper
- 4 lemon wedges

Instructions:
- Peel shrimp and butterfly them.

- Place shrimp in marinade: 2 tbsp olive oil, lemon, garlic powder. Marinade anywhere from 15 minutes to hours.

- Heat 2 tbsp of oil in a pan on medium to high

heat.

- Add shrimp and cook each side for 2-3 minutes. Drizzle with 1 Tablespoon of olive oil.

- Top with salt, pepper, and red pepper flakes.

CITRUS SHRIMP

Ingredients:

- 3/4 lbs peeled and deveined medium shrimp
- 1/2 Tbsp almond meal
- 2 Tbsp orange juice, fresh squeezed
- 1/2 Tbsp rice vinegar
- 1 Tbsp diced chili
- 1 Tbsp olive oil
- 1/2 Tbsp fresh ginger, minced
- 2 garlic cloves, minced

Instructions:

- In a large nonstick skillet, heat the oil. Saute the shrimp until just pink, about 2-3 minutes.
- Add the garlic and cook stirring constantly, about 30 seconds. With a slotted spoon transfer the shrimp to a platter and keep them warm.
- In the skillet, combine the broth, lemon juice, 1/4 cup of the parsley, the salt and pepper; and bring it to a boil. Boil uncovered, until the sauce is reduced by half.
- Spoon the sauce over the shrimp. Serve garnished with the lemon wedges and sprinkled with the remaining tablespoon of parsley.

GARLIC SHRIMP

Ingredients:
- 4-5 tbsp olive oil
- 4 garlic cloves, minced
- 1 tbsp red pepper flakes
- 1 tbsp smoked paprika
- 1 lb medium shrimp, peeled and deveined
- 2 tbsp fresh lime juice
- 2 tsp jerez sherry
- salt and pepper to taste

Instructions:

- Place shrimp in a bowl and toss with almond powder. Make sure shrimp is evenly coated.

- In a small bowl whisk together orange juice, rice vinegar and chili Heat olive oil in a large non-stick skillet over medium-high heat.

- Add ginger and garlic. Stir until garlic becomes fragrant.

- Add shrimp and cook for 3 minutes. Add in sauce and cook for an additional 2 minutes. Remove shrimp with a slotted spoon.

- Continue stirring sauce for another 2-4 minutes until it thickens. Drizzle over shrimp. Serve on top of baby spinach or fried cauliflower rice.

SHRIMP CAKES

Ingredients:

- 2 cups of small prawns
- 2 eggs
- fresh chives
- 1/2 tsp spicy chili powder
- 1/2 tsp ground coriander
- 1/2 tsp garlic powder
- shredded coconut
- 1/2 tbsp coconut flour

Instructions:

- In a saute pan over medium heat, warm the olive oil.
- Add the garlic, red pepper flakes and paprika and saute for 1 minute until fragrant.
- Increase the heat to high, add the shrimp, lime juice and sherry, stir well, and saute until the shrimp.
- Season with salt and black pepper.

SHRIMP SPINACH

Ingredients:
- 2 tablespoons olive oil
- 1 diced yellow onion
- 1 cup green beans
- 2 cloves garlic minced
- 1 tsp chili powder
- Juice of 1 lime
- 1 lb shrimp
- 6 oz baby spinach
- salt and pepper to taste

Instructions:

- Chop the shrimp, Next, mix in the spices, chives, 1 egg and the coconut flour. Set up 2 bowls, 1 with shredded coconut and the other with the 2nd egg, whisked.

- Form cakes of the shrimp mix - cover them with the whisked egg and then with shredded coconut.

- Cook them in coconut oil on both sides until brown.

- Serve with vegetables of your choice, or fried cauliflower rice.

HERBED SALMON

Ingredients:
- 4 garlic cloves
- 1 tsp dried Herbs de Provence
- 1 tsp red wine vinegar
- 1 tsp olive oil
- 2 tbsp mustard powder
- olive oil spray
- 4 wild salmon filets, 1" thick (if frozen, thaw first)
- salt and fresh ground pepper to taste
- 4 lemon wedges for serving

Instructions:

- In a mini food processor, or using a mortar and pestle, mash garlic with the herbs, vinegar, oil, and mustard until it becomes a paste. Set aside.

- Season salmon with a pinch of low sodium salt and fresh pepper. Heat a grill or grill pan over high heat until hot.

- Spray the pan lightly with oil and reduce the heat to medium-low. Place the salmon on the hot grill pan and cook without moving for 5 minutes.

- Turn and cook the other side for an additional 3-4 minutes spooning on half of the garlic herb mustard sauce.

- Turn and cook for 1 more minute, spooning the other side of the fish with remaining sauce. Turn once again and let the fish finish cooking for about one more minute.

- Serve with a green salad and paleo dressing

HALIBUT SOUP

Ingredients:
- 1 tsp olive oil
- 2 chopped shallots
- 2 cloves of garlic
- 3 medium diced tomatoes
- 4 oz cup of white wine
- 1 cup clam juice
- 2 cups vegetable stock
- 3/4 lb halibut filet, skin removed cut into large pieces
- 1 dozen small clams
- pinch of saffron
- 1/4 cup fresh chopped parsley

Instructions:
- Add olive oil to a large heavy pot; over medium heat saute shallots and garlic until translucent.

- Add the tomatoes, wine, clam juice and the bone from the halibut if you have one. Add vegetable stock, saffron, fresh thyme and stir.

- Add the clams; cover and cook for 2

minutes, add the fish and cook for an additional 3 minutes, or until the shrimp turns pink and the clams open.

TERIYAKI SALMON

Ingredients:
- 3 tbsp low-sodium soy sauce
- 3 tbsp mirin
- 3 tbsp sake
- Stevia to taste
- 1 lb fresh wild salmon filet, cut in 4 pieces
- 2 tsp cooking oil

Instructions:
- Combine the soy sauce, mirin, sake, and stevia in a resealable bag. Add the salmon and mix to coat. Refrigerate for 1 hour or up to 8 hours.

- Remove salmon, reserving the marinade. Heat a frying pan or saute pan over medium-high heat. When hot, swirl in the oil.

- Sear salmon, 2 minutes per side. Turn heat to low and pour in the reserved marinade. Cover and cook for 4 to 5 minutes, until cooked through.

- Serve with cauliflower rice

SHRIMP CAKES

Ingredients:
- 1 lb shrimp, peeled and deveined
- 1 large jalapeno, seeded and minced
- 1 garlic clove, minced
- 3 medium scallions, chopped
- 2 tablespoons fresh cilantro, chopped
- 1/4 teaspoon salt
- 1/8 teaspoon fresh ground black pepper
- 1 tablespoon almond flour

For topping:
- 4 lime wedges
- 1/2 medium avocado, sliced thin

Instructions:
- Dry shrimp well with a paper towel then place the shrimp in the food processor along with jalapeno and garlic then pulse a few times until almost pasty.

- Combine the shrimp in a large bowl with remaining ingredients and mix well to combine.

- Using rubber gloves (easier with gloves), form shrimp into 4 patties.

- Heat a non-stick skillet over medium heat and spray with oil. Add the shrimp cakes to the heated grill and cook for 4 minutes without disturbing, then gently flip and cook for an additional 4 minutes.

- Serve with fresh lime juice and celeriac mash.

TASTY SEARED SCAMPI

Ingredients:
- 2 tsp olive oil
- 1 1/2 lbs shrimp, peeled and deveined
- 1/4 tsp salt
- 1/4 tsp ground black pepper
- 1/4 tsp crushed red pepper
- 2 tbsp dry parsley
- lemon wedges

Instructions:
- Heat 1 tsp oil in a 12 inch skillet over high heat until smoking.Meanwhile, toss shrimp with low sodium salt and pepper.

- Add half of the shrimp to the pan in a single layer and cook until the edges turn pink, about 1 minute.

- Remove pan from heat, flip shrimp using tongs and let it stand about 30 seconds until all of the shrimp is opaque except for the center.

- Transfer to a plate and repeat with the second batch and the remaining teaspoon of oil. After the second batch has stood off the heat, add the first batch to the pan and toss to combine.

- Cover the skillet and let the shrimp stand for 1 - 2 minutes. Serve immediately with a green salad and lemon wedges.

LIGHT SLAW

Ingredients:
- 1/2 head of cabbage (mix purple and white)
- 3 or 4 carrots
- 1 onion
- 3 tablespoons walnut oil
- 1 egg beaten
- Stevia to taste
- 2 Tbsp. fresh lemon juice
- pepper to taste

Instructions:
- Grate cabbage, carrots and onion and mix together.

- Make dressing by mixing beaten egg, walnut oil, lemon juice, and seasonings.

- Chill and serve.

TURKEY EASTERN STYLE

Ingredients:

For the salad:

- 2 cups grilled turkey, chopped
- 6 baby bok choy, grilled & chopped
- 2 green onions, chopped
- 1/4 cup cilantro, chopped
- 1 Tbsp sesame seeds

For the dressing:

- 1 tbsp fresh ginger, chopped
- 1 tbsp coconut cream
- 1 tbsp fish sauce
- 1 tbsp sesame oil
- 1 tbsp fresh lime juice
- 1 tsp stevia powder or to taste

Instructions:

- Combine all of the salad ingredients until well mixed.

- Add all of the ingredients for the dressing into a blender or food processor, and blend until mostly smooth.

- Pour the dressing over the salad and toss lightly until coated.

- Garnish with more sesame seeds if desired.

MEDITERRANEAN TURKEY SALAD

Ingredients:

- 1 roasted turkey
- 1/2 cup of olive oil
- 1/4 cup fresh cilantro, chopped
- 1 head of romaine or butter lettuce
- 1 red onion, diced
- 1 lemon, juiced
- salt and pepper as desired

Instructions:

- Shred the turkey with your hands or chop up and put it in a big bowl.
- Add the oil, red onion, cilantro, lemon, salt and pepper.
- Mix well and serve on a lettuce boat.

LIGHT TURKEY DIVINE

Ingredients:

- 2/3 cup fresh lime juice
- 1/3 cup fish sauce
- Stevia to taste

- 3/4 cup chicken stock low sodium
- 1 1/2 pounds ground turkey
- 1 cup thinly sliced green onions
- 3/4 cup thinly sliced shallots
- 3 tbsp minced lemongrass
- 1 tbsp thinly sliced Serrano chili
- 1/2 cup chopped cilantro leaves
- 1/3 cup chopped mint leaves
- Salt to taste
- 1 head lettuce

Instructions:

- Whisk together lime juice, fish sauce, honey and chili-garlic sauce. Set aside.

- Warm chicken stock in a medium heavy-bottomed pot until simmering. Add ground turkey and simmer until cooked through for 6 to 8 minutes. Add green onion, shallot, lemongrass and chilies, stirring to combine. Continue cooking until shallots turn translucent, stirring occasionally (about 4 minutes). Remove from the heat and drain off any liquid in the pot.

- Stir in lime juice-fish sauce mixture, cilantro and mint. Season to taste with low sodium salt (not much is needed if any).

CHICKEN BASIL AVOCADO SALAD

Ingredients:
- 2 boneless, skinless chicken breasts (cooked and shredded)
- 1/2 cup fresh basil leaves, stems removed
- 1 cup sliced cherry tomatoes
- 1 large ripe avocado, pit and skin removed
- 2 tbsp extra virgin olive oil
- 1/2 tsp salt to taste
- 1/8 tsp ground black pepper

Instructions:

- Place the cooked shredded chicken in a medium sized mixing bowl.

- Place the basil, avocado, olive oil, low sodium salt and ground black pepper in a food processor and blend until smooth. You may need to scrape the sides a couple times to incorporate.

- Pour the avocado and basil mixture into the mixing bowl with the shredded chicken and tomatoes and toss well to coat.

- Taste and add additional low sodium salt and ground black pepper if desired. Keep in the fridge until ready to serve

ZUCCHINI CASSEROLE

Ingredients:
- 3 large zucchini
- 1/2 red onion, chopped
- 1/2 cup mushrooms
- 5 eggs
- 1 tsp salt
- ground black pepper, to taste

Instructions:
- Preheat the oven to 375 degrees F. Grate all of the zucchini and put into a large bowl.

- In a separate bowl, beat the eggs with low sodium salt and pepper.Combine all of the ingredients in the large bowl and mix together.

- Heat 1/2 tablespoon of olive oil in the skillet over medium heat. Add the zucchini mixture into the pan. Cover and cook for about 5 minutes until the eggs start to set on the bottom.

- Transfer to the oven and bake for 12-15 minutes, until the eggs are firm. Remove and let rest for 5-10 minutes, then serve.

BLUEBERRY NUT CASSEROLE

Ingredients:
- 2 cups frozen blueberries
- 5 eggs
- 1 cup almond milk
- Stevia to taste
- 1 tsp vanilla extract
- 1 tsp cinnamon
- Pinch of nutmeg

Instructions:
- Preheat the oven to 350 degrees F. Grease an 8x8-inch baking dish with coconut oil spray. Place the nut crust and blueberries into the dish.

- Whisk together the eggs, almond milk, stevia, vanilla, and cinnamon in a medium bowl.

- Pour the egg mixture over the crust and blueberries. Lightly stir to coat.

- Bake for 35-45 minutes. Remove from the oven and allow the casserole to rest for 15 minutes before serving.

LIGHT CHICKEN SALAD

Ingredients:

Salad:
- 4 cups cabbage, finely shredded
- 1 cup carrot, julienned
- 1/4 cup scallions, trimmed and julienned
- 1/4 cup radishes, julienned
- 1/4 cup fresh cilantro, chopped
- 1/4 cup fresh mint, chopped
- 2 cups cooked organic chicken

Vinaigrette:
- 2 tablespoons coconut or rice vinegar
- 2 tablespoons sesame oil
- juice of 1/2 a lime
- 1 chipotle pepper
- 1 clove garlic, crushed
- 1 teaspoon fresh ginger, grated

Instructions:

- Combine cabbage, carrots, scallions and radishes. Top with chicken, cilantro and mint and set aside.

- Combine the vinaigrette ingredients. Taste to see if it needs any adjustments.

- Drizzle salad with vinaigrette & enjoy.

SPINACH OMELET

Ingredients:

- 2 eggs
- 1 1/2 cups raw spinach
- 1 tbsp coconut oil, about 1 tbsp
- 1/3 cup tomatoes and onion salsa
- 1 tbsp fresh cilantro

Instructions:

- Melt coconut oil on medium in a frying pan. Add spinach, cook until mostly wilted. Beat eggs and add to pan.

- Flip once the egg sets around the edge. When it's almost done add the salsa on top just to warm it. Move to plate and add cilantro. Serves one.

BLUEBERRY OMELET

Ingredients:

- 2 eggs
- 1 tsp. vanilla extract
- coconut oil
- 1/2 cup blueberries
- Stevia to taste

Instructions:

- Lightly beat two eggs and vanilla extract in a bowl. Heat a non-stick pan.

- While the pan is heating, heat half the blueberries in a saucepan until juices flow.
- Add coconut oil to a non-stick pan and coat evenly. When thoroughly heated, add egg mixture. Swish once and let sit.
- When eggs are about 70% settled, swish again. There should be a nice crispy layer around the side of the pan.
- When it starts to separate from the side, add fresh and cooked blueberries to omelet, reserving a few for garnish.
- Use a fork to help fold the omelet over. Slide on to plate, top with reserved blueberry filling, and enjoy

LETTUCE MUSHROOMS WRAPS

Ingredients:
- 8 oz skinless, boneless chicken or turkey ground
- 1/4 cup water chestnuts, chopped
- 1/4 cup dried shiitake mushrooms
- 1 tbsp soy sauce
- 1 1/2 tsp sesame oil
- 1 tsp rice wine or dry sherry
- 1/2 tsp stevia
- freshly ground white pepper, to taste
- 2 cloves garlic, finely chopped
- 6 large iceberg lettuce leaves, rinsed
- 2 tbsp diced scallions

Instructions:

- Place mushrooms in hot water to soften for a few minutes. Remove stems and chop fine.

- Combine all sauces and dry ingredients in a bowl. Combine ground chicken mushrooms and water chestnuts into a bowl. Pour over chicken; toss. Let marinate for 15 minutes.

- Heat remaining sesame oil in a wok or skillet over high heat. Add garlic; cook until golden, about 10 seconds.

- Add chicken mixture; stir fry until browned, breaking the chicken up as it cooks, about 4-5 minutes.

- To serve, spoon 1/4 cup of the mixture into each lettuce leaf. Garnish with scallions.

STEAK SKEWERS

Ingredients:
- 1 1/2 lbs sliced flank steak
- 1 1/2 cups reduced sodium soy sauce
- 2 cloves minced garlic
- 1 tsp fresh ginger
- 1 tsp sesame oil
- Juice of 1 lime

Instructions:
- Soak wooden skewers in water. Marinate the steak/venison in all the ingredients for about 1

hour or more.

- Thread the sliced steak onto the skewers.

- Heat your grill or grill pan to high heat; when hot grill a few minutes on each side until browned and cooked though.

- Use marinade as dipping sauce.

AVOCADO STUFFED WITH TUNA

Ingredients:
- 1 medium avocado
- 2 tins tuna
- 2 tbsp chopped red onion
- Juice of 1 lime
- 1 tbsp chopped cilantro
- 1 tsp olive oil
- salt and pepper to taste

Instructions:

- In a medium bowl, combine onion, lime juice, olive oil, cilantro salt and pepper. Add crab meat and toss well.

- Cut the avocado open, remove the pit and spoon out the avocado. Cut into large chunks and add to tuna.

- Mix carefully, not to mash the avocado. Spoon

back into avocado shells and enjoy!

AVOCADO AND PEACH SALSA

Ingredients:
- 1 peach, peeled and diced
- 1 avocado, peeled and diced
- 1 plum tomato, diced
- 1 clove garlic, minced
- 1/4 cup chopped fresh cilantro
- 2 tbsp fresh lime juice
- 1/4 cup chopped red onion
- 1 tbsp olive oil
- Salt and fresh pepper to taste

Instructions:
- Combine all the ingredients and let it marinate in the refrigerator 30 minutes before serving.

BAKED CRISPY SWEET POTATO FRIES

Ingredients:
- 1 sweet potato, cut into 1/4" fries
- 2 tsp olive oil
- Salt to taste
- Ground paprika
- Ground chili
- garlic powder

Instructions:
- Preheat the oven to 425°F.

- In a medium bowl, toss sweet potatoes with olive oil, low sodium salt, paprika, garlic powder and chili powder.

- Spread potatoes on a baking sheet. Avoid crowding so potatoes get crisp. Bake for 15 minutes.

- Turn and bake for an additional 10-15 minutes. Ovens may vary so keep an eye on them and be sure to cut all the potatoes the same size to ensure even cooking.

BAKED SALMON CAKES WITH RED PEPPER LIME SAUCE

Ingredients:
- 9 oz salmon flakes
- 1 whole egg + 1 egg white, beaten
- 2 finely chopped scallions
- 2 tbsp finely chopped red bell pepper
- 1 tbsp low fat paleo mayo
- 2 tbsp fresh cilantro (or parsley)
- 1/2 lime, juiced
- salt and pepper to taste

Instructions:

- In a large bowl, combine eggs, scallions, pepper, mayo, cilantro, lime juice, salt and pepper. Mix well, then fold in fish, careful not to over mix gently into patties using a 1/2 cup measuring cup.

- Chill in the refrigerator at least 1/2 hour before baking.

- Preheat the oven to 400°F. Grease a baking sheet with cooking spray.

- Bake about 8-10 minutes on each side, until nicely browned.

- Drizzle lime juice over cakes and serve.

BAKED PRAWN CAKES

Ingredients:
- 1/2 lb frozen or fresh prawns
- salt, to taste
- olive oil cooking spray
- 1 tbsp olive oil
- salt and freshly ground black pepper
- 3/4 cup small-diced red onion
- 1 1/2 cups small-diced celery
- 1/2 cup small-diced red bell pepper
- 1/2 cup small-diced yellow bell pepper
- 1/4 cup minced fresh flat-leaf parsley
- 1 large egg, lightly beaten
- 3 large egg whites, lightly beaten
- 2 tsp mustard

Instructions:

- Season prawns with low sodium salt. Heat a large saute pan over medium- high heat; when hot lightly spray with oil and add the salmon. Cook until browned on one side, Set aside on a dish to cool.

- Add the olive oil to the pan, then add the onion, celery, red and yellow bell peppers, parsley, 1/2 teaspoon low sodium salt, and 1/2 teaspoon pepper in a large saute pan over medium-low heat and cook until the vegetables are soft, approximately 18 to 20 minutes. Set aside to cool to room temperature. Cut large chunks of prawn into a large bowl. Add the mustard, and eggs.

- Add the vegetable mixture and mix well. Cover and chill in the refrigerator for 30 minutes, this will make them easier to shape and become less sticky.

- Preheat the oven to 400°F. Spray a non-stick baking sheet with cooking spray. Shape the batter into 15 (scant 1/4 cup each) cakes and place on a prepared baking sheet.

- Bake about 10 to 12 minutes on each side, or until golden brown.

FRIES WITH GARLIC AIOLI

Ingredients:
- 4 medium sweet potatoes
- 2 tsp olive oil
- 1 tbsp herbs de provence
- 1/4 tsp oregano
- 1 tsp smoked paprika
- 1/4 tsp chili powder
- 1/4 tsp onion powder
- 1/4 tsp garlic powder
- 1/4 tsp fresh cracked pepper
- fresh lime zest

Skinny Garlic Aioli:
- 2 paleo mayo
- 1 clove garlic, crushed

Instructions:

- Preheat the oven to 400°F. Line the baking sheet with foil for easy clean-up.

- Lightly coat with cooking spray. Cut each potato lengthwise into 1/4 inch slices; cut each slice into 1/4 inch fries. In a large bowl, combine cut potatoes and oil; toss well. Add rosemary, thyme, garlic and seasoning. Toss to coat.

- Place in a single layer on a lightly greased baking sheet. Bake for about 25 minutes or until tender crisp, turning once halfway through. Serve with garlic aioli.

BAKED PLANTAINS

Ingredients:

- 3 medium green plantains
- 2 tsp olive oil
- salt

Lemon Garlic Dipping Sauce:

- 1/3 cup lemon juice
- 2 tsp olive oil
- 1 large clove garlic, minced
- A pinch of oregano
- A pinch of low sodium salt and pepper
- 1/2 tsp cumin

Instructions:

- Preheat the oven to 400°. Spray baking sheet

with cooking spray.

- Peel plantains and slice into 1/2 thick slices. Place in a bowl and toss with oil and salt. Arrange slices on the baking sheet. Lightly coat with a little more oil spray on top and bake for 10 minutes or until slightly brown on the bottom. Remove from the oven.

- Lightly re-spray the baking sheet and place the plantains brown side up onto the baking sheet. Lightly spray the top and bake for another 15 minutes until golden brown and crispy.

- Heat a small saucepan on low flame, when hot add oil. Saute garlic on low for about 2 minutes, do not brown. Add lemon juice, oregano, cumin, salt and pepper and let it come to a boil. Set aside to cool to room temperature.

TURKEY CROQUETTES

Ingredients:
- 12 oz cooked chopped turkey breast
- 1/2 head Steamed cauliflower
- 2 tsp olive oil
- 3 cloves garlic
- 1 medium onion, chopped
- 1/2 cup parsley, chopped
- salt and pepper
- 1 egg, beaten
- 2 tbsp almond flour

Instructions:

- In a large bowl, mash cauliflower with 1/4 cup broth, low sodium salt and pepper. Set aside.

- Saute garlic, and onions in oil on low heat. Add parsley, low sodium salt and pepper and cook until soft, about 2-3 minutes. Add turkey, and remaining broth, mix well and shut heat off.

- Add turkey to mashed cauliflower and use your clean hands to mix well. Use some almond flour to bind. Taste for low sodium salt and adjust if needed.

- Preheat the oven to 450°F. Measure 1/4 cup of mixture then form into croquettes. Place on waxed paper. Repeat with remaining mixture.

- Dip each croquette in egg wash, and place on a parchment lined cookie sheet for easy cleanup.

Spray generously with olive oil spray .Bake in the oven for about 15 minutes, or until golden.

ZESTY SHRIMP

Ingredients:

For the Shrimp:
- 1 lb large shrimp , shelled and deveined
- 2 tbsp olive oil
- 2 tbsp lemon juice +1 tsp garlic powder mixed together
- 3 cups shredded iceberg lettuce
- 1 cup shredded purple cabbage
- 4 tbsp scallions, chopped

Instructions:
- Combine lettuce and cabbage and divide between four plates. Set aside.Heat a large skillet or wok on high heat, when hot add oil. When oil is hot add the shrimp to a hot pan and cook tossing a few times until cooked through, about 3 minutes.
- Remove from the pan and pour lemon juice and garlic powder mix over the shrimp.Place shrimp on lettuce and top with scallions.

AVOCADO, CUCUMBER & TOMATO SALAD

Ingredients:
- 1 seedless cucumber, peeled and diced
- 2 medium ripe tomatoes, diced
- 2 avocados, diced

- 2 tbsp red onion, minced
- 2 tbsp cilantro, minced
- 2 limes, juice of
- salt and fresh pepper

Instructions:

- Combine all the ingredients and season with salt and pepper to taste.

SASHIMI CUCUMBER CUPS

Ingredients:

- 8 oz fresh raw fish filet finely sliced
- 1 medium seeded tomato, finely diced
- 1 tbsp chopped cilantro
- 1 tbsp minced red onion
- 1/2 jalapeno, minced
- 1/4 yellow bell pepper, finely diced
- 1/2 tbsp olive oil
- 3 tbsp fresh lime, (1 or 2 limes)
- Low sodium salt and freshly ground black pepper, as needed
- 2 large cucumbers (sliced to 1/2-inch-thick slices)
- fresh cilantro for garnishing

Instructions:

- In a medium bowl, combine the sea bass, tomato, onion, chopped cilantro, jalapeno, bell pepper, oil

- Add the lime juice and toss to coat the fish.

Season with low sodium salt and pepper. Cover and marinate in the refrigerator for at least 1 hour depending on the size of the fish cubes, stirring occasionally.

- Trim the cucumber slices with a round cutter to remove the rind. With a melon baller, scoop out a shallow pocket in the middle of the cucumber slices—do not cut all the way through the slice.

- Just before serving, fill the cucumber cups with the sashimi.

CALAMARI LEMON SALAD SURPRISE

Ingredients:
- 1/4 cup red onion, minced
- 1/2 cup celery, chopped
- 1/2 cup roasted red peppers, chopped
- 1/4 cup fresh parsley, minced
- 1 clove garlic, sliced
- 1 1/2 lemons
- 1 1/4 tsp red wine vinegar
- salt and pepper to taste
- 1 lb fresh squid, tube and tentacles cleaned

Instructions:
- Rinse squid and slice tubes into 1/2 inch rings. Leave the tentacles whole and set aside. Prepare a bowl of water with ice.

- In a medium bowl combine onion, garlic, celery, red peppers, parsley, lemon juice, vinegar, low sodium salt and fresh pepper.

- Bring a medium pot filled with water and a pinch of salt to a boil. Add calamari all at once and cook until tender yet cooked. Drain and add to the ice bath until cool, 4 - 5 minutes.

- Combine squid with the salad and toss well. Cover and refrigerate at least an hour.

LOBSTER SALAD

Ingredients:
- 12 oz cooked, chilled lobster meat
- 1 cup grape tomatoes, sliced in half
- 1 tbsp chopped chives
- juice of 1 large lemon
- 4 tsp olive oil
- salt and pepper to taste
- 8 lettuce leaves, rinsed and dried

Instructions:
- Chop chilled lobster meat from tails and claws into large bite sized chunks; add to the bowl. Add tomatoes, chives, lemon juice, olive oil, and low sodium salt and fresh cracked pepper to taste; toss to combine.

- Place lettuce leaves on two plates. Top each

plate with lobster salad and enjoy!

TURKEY AND ZUCCHINI YAKITORI

Ingredients:
- 1/2 cup low sodium soy sauce gluten free
- 4 drops tsp stevia
- 1 garlic clove, crushed
- 1 lb turkey breast diced
- 5 large green onions, cut 1-inch-long
- 1 medium zucchini, sliced into 1/2-inch thick rings

Instructions:
- Bring low sodium soy sauce, stevia and crushed garlic to a boil in a medium-sized saucepan, and cook over medium heat for about 5 minutes. Set aside to cool.

- Cut the turkey into 1-inch pieces and place in a ziplock bag; pour half of the marinade over. Place the zucchini in a second large ziplock bag and pour the remaining marinade over the zucchini. Refrigerate for at least 30 minutes.

- Thread the turkey onto skewers, alternating with green onion so that each stick has 3 cubes of chicken and two pieces of green onion.

- Thread the zucchini onto skewers, alternating with remaining green onion, reserving the marinade for basting.

- Preheat the grill or a grill pan over medium-high heat. When hot, spray with oil then reduce heat to medium; grill the zucchini and skewer about 5 to 6 minutes on each side brushing both sides of the skewers with the yakitori sauce during the last few minutes of cooking time.

GRILLED PRAWN KEBABS

Ingredients:

- 32 jumbo raw tiger prawns, peeled and deveined
- 2 cloves garlic, crushed
- 3 large limes thinly sliced
- olive oil cooking spray
- 1 tsp low sodium salt
- 1 1/2 tsp ground cumin
- 1/4 cup chopped fresh cilantro, divided
- 1 lime cut into 8 wedges

Instructions:

- Heat the grill on medium heat and spray the grates with oil. Season the prawns with garlic, cumin, low sodium salt and half of the cilantro in a medium bowl.

- Beginning and ending with shrimp, thread the shrimp and folded lime slices onto 8 pairs of parallel skewers to make 8 kebabs total.

- Grill the prawns, turning occasionally, until opaque throughout, about 1 to 2 minutes on each side. Top with remaining cilantro and fresh squeezed lime juice before serving.

SPLENDID GUACAMOLE

Ingredients:
- 3 medium avocados, halved
- 1 lime, juiced
- 1/3 cup white onion, minced
- 1 small clove garlic, smashed
- 1 tbsp chopped cilantro
- salt and fresh pepper, to taste

Instructions:
- Place the pulp from the avocados in a medium bowl and slightly mash with a fork or a potato masher leaving some large chunks.

- Add lime juice, low sodium salt, pepper, cilantro, onion, garlic and mix thoroughly.

PUMPKIN AVOCADO SALAD

Ingredients:
- 2 tbsp red onion, chopped
- 2 tbsp lime juice
- 2 medium avocados, diced
- 2 cups cooked pumpkin, diced
- 2 tbsp chopped cilantro
- salt and pepper to taste

Instructions:
- In a small bowl combine onion, lime juice and low sodium salt.

- In a medium bowl, combine avocados, pumpkin, and cilantro. Toss with lime juice and onions and serve immediately.

TURKEY KEBABS

Ingredients:
- 20 oz lean ground turkey
- 1 small onion, minced
- 2 cloves garlic, minced
- 1/4 cup fresh parsley, chopped
- 1/4 tsp allspice
- 1/4 tsp coriander
- 1/4 tsp paprika
- 1/4 tsp chili powder
- Low sodium salt and fresh pepper (to taste)

Instructions:
- In a large bowl combine the ground turkey, onion, garlic, parsley, spices, low sodium salt and pepper until evenly blended.

- Divide into a heaping 1/4 cup portion so you get 12; roll into log shaped ovals. Place on a cookie sheet and refrigerate for at least 30 minutes. If using wooden skewers, soak in water at least 30 minutes before grilling.

- When ready to eat, preheat the grill to high heat. Carefully insert the skewer through the formed meat.

- Grill for 10 to 15 minutes on indirect heat turning occasionally, until meat is no longer pink.

PUNCHY TOMATO SALSA

Ingredients:
- 4 medium ripe tomatoes, chopped
- 1/4 cup finely chopped white onion
- 2 chili peppers, mild or hot, seeded and finely chopped
- 2 tbsp chopped bell pepper
- 1 clove garlic, minced
- 1/4 cup finely chopped fresh cilantro leaves
- 2 tbsp fresh lime juice
- salt and pepper to taste

Instructions:
- In a bowl combine all ingredients. Let it marinate in the refrigerator for at least an hour for best results.

TOMATO SALSA

Ingredients:
- 3 medium tomatoes, cored and quartered
- 1 jalapeno, stem removed and roasted
- 3-4 small cloves garlic
- 2 tbsp cilantro
- 3-4 tbsp water
- 1 tsp olive oil
- salt to taste

Instructions:
- In a blender, add tomatoes, jalapeno, garlic, cilantro and water and pulse a few times until

completely smooth.

- Add oil to a deep skillet, then pour in tomatoes. Season with salt and simmer uncovered, stirring occasionally, 20 to 25 minutes.

SHRIMP COCKTAIL

Ingredients:
- 1/4 cup chopped red onion
- 2 small limes, squeezed
- 1 tsp olive oil
- 1 lb large cooked shrimp, peeled and deveined
- 1 medium avocado, diced into chunks
- 1 medium tomato, diced
- 1 cup diced English cucumber, not peeled
- 1 serrano pepper, seeds removed and minced
- 2 tbsp chopped cilantro, plus more for garnish
- salt and pepper to taste
- lime wedges for serving
- 2 1/4 cups shredded iceberg lettuce

Instructions:
- In a small bowl combine red onion, lime juice, olive oil, pinch of salt and pepper. Let them marinate for at least 5 minutes to mellow the flavor of the onion.

- In a large bowl combine shrimp, avocado, tomato, cucumber, and serrano pepper. Combine all the ingredients together, add cilantro and gently toss. Adjust low sodium salt and pepper to taste.

- Fill wine glasses with shredded lettuce. Top each with 1/2 cup shrimp salad and garnish with a sprig of cilantro. Serve with a wedge of lime.

CRISPY CHICKEN WINGS

Ingredients:
- 3 lbs chicken wings
- 1/4 cup white vinegar
- 2 tbsp oregano
- 4 tsp paprika
- 1 tbsp garlic powder
- 1 tbsp chili powder
- Low sodium salt and fresh pepper
- 2 celery stalks, sliced into strips
- 2 carrots, peeled and sliced into strips

Instructions:

- In a large bowl combine chicken, vinegar, oregano, paprika, garlic powder, chili powder salt and pepper. Mix well and let marinate for 30 minutes.

- Place wings on a broiler rack and broil on low, about 8 inches from the flame for about 10-12 minutes on each side.

- While chicken cooks, heat the remaining

hot sauce until warm. Toss the hot sauce with the chicken and arrange on a platter. Serve with celery and carrot strips.

PRAWN SALSA

Ingredients:
- 16 oz cooked peeled prawns diced in large chunks
- 4 vine ripe tomatoes, diced fine
- 6 tbsp red onion, finely diced
- 2 tbsp minced cilantro
- 2 limes, juice of (or more to taste)
- 1/2 tsp salt

Instructions:
- Combine diced onions, tomatoes, salt and lime juice in a non-reactive bowl and let it sit about 5 minutes.
- Combine the remaining ingredients in a large bowl. Refrigerate and let the flavors combine at least an hour before serving.

DIVINE JUICY TUNA SASHIMI

Ingredients:
- 8 oz sushi grade tuna, finely chopped
- 2 tsp pure sesame oil
- 1 tsp rice wine
- 2 tsp fresh lime juice
- 2 tsp low sodium gluten free soy sauce

- 1 ripe, firm avocado, diced
- 1 tsp black and white sesame seeds

Instructions:

- Combine sesame oil, lime juice, and soy sauce.
- Pour over tuna and mix. Add chives and gently combine tuna with diced avocado, refrigerate until ready to serve. top with sesame seeds.

STEAMED MUSSELS WITH FRESH BASIL

Ingredients:

- 2 dozen mussels
- 2 tsp olive oil
- 3 cloves garlic, sliced
- 2 tbsp fresh herbs such as basil
- 1 tbsp white wine
- 1/4 cup water

Instructions:

- Heat a large pot on high heat. Add oil. When hot, add garlic and cook until golden.

- Add wine, water and mussels and cover tightly, reduce to medium-low heat.

- Cook for 5 to 10 minutes, or until the shells open. Do not overcook or the mussels will become rubbery.

- Transfer with a slotted spoon to a large bowl and pour the liquid through a strainer over the clams. Top with fresh herbs and enjoy.

SUMMER TUNA AND AVOCADO SALAD

Ingredients:
- 2 water canned tuna
- 1 pint grape tomatoes, cut in half
- 1 avocado, diced
- 2 hot peppers such as serrano or jalapenos, diced
- 1/3 cup chopped red onion
- 2 limes, juice of (or more to taste)
- 1 tsp olive oil
- 2 tbsp chopped cilantro
- salt and fresh pepper to taste

Instructions:
- In a small bowl combine red onion, lime juice, olive oil, pinch of low sodium salt and pepper. Let them marinate for at least 5 minutes to mellow the flavor of the onion.
- In a large bowl combine tuna, avocado, tomatoes, hot pepper Combine all the ingredients together, add cilantro and gently toss. Adjust lime juice, low sodium salt and pepper to taste.

ZESTY SALMON AND AVOCADO SALAD

Ingredients:
- 3 cups Cubed steamed salmon
- 1 medium tomato, diced

- 1 avocado, diced
- 1 jalapeno, seeds removed, diced fine
- 1/4 cup chopped red onion
- 2 limes, juice
- 1 tsp olive oil
- 1 tbsp chopped cilantro
- salt and fresh pepper to taste

Instructions:

- In a small bowl combine red onion, lime juice, olive oil, pinch of low sodium salt and pepper. Let them marinate for at least 5 minutes to mellow the flavor of the onion.

- In a large bowl combine salmon, avocado, tomato, jalapeno. Combine all the ingredients together, add cilantro and gently toss. Adjust salt and pepper to taste.

MEDITERRANEAN R OMELET WITH FENNEL AND DILL

Ingredients:
- 2 tablespoons olive oil, divided
- 2 cups thinly sliced fresh fennel bulb, fronds chopped and reserved
- 8 cherry tomatoes
- 5 large eggs, beaten salt and pepper
- 1 1/2 tablespoons chopped fresh dill

Instructions:
- Add remaining oil to the same skillet; heat over medium-high heat.

- Add beaten eggs and cook until eggs are just set in center, tilting skillet and lifting edges of omelet with spatula to let uncooked portion flow underneath, about 3 minutes.

- Top with fennel mixture. Sprinkle dill over.Using spatula, fold uncovered half of omelet over; slide onto plate.

- Garnish with chopped fennel and serve.

VEGGIE OMELET

Ingredients:

- 3 eggs, beaten
- 1 carrot, matchstick cut
- 3 scallions, diagonal sliced
- 1 handful tiny broccoli florets or leftover veggies
- Leftover cooked turkey
- Salt

Instructions:

- Heat oil in a wok or large cast iron skillet over medium heat, until hot enough to sizzle a drop of water.

- Add broccoli and carrots, stir fry 2 min. until soft.

- Add cooked turkey, stir fry 1 min. until heated through. Add scallions and eggs, scramble. Add salt to taste. Serve.

BASIL TURKEY WITH ROASTED TOMATOES

Ingredients:
- 2 turkey breasts
- 1 cup mushrooms, chopped
- 1/2 medium onion, chopped
- 1-2 tbsp extra virgin olive oil
- 1/2 cup thinly sliced fresh basil
- low sodium salt and pepper, to taste
- 1 pint cherry tomatoes
- Stevia to taste
- Fresh parsley, for garnish

Instructions:
- Preheat the oven to 400 degrees F. Place the tomatoes on a baking sheet and drizzle with olive oil and stevia. Sprinkle with low sodium salt and pepper and toss to coat evenly. Bake for 15-20 minutes until soft.

- While the tomatoes are roasting, heat one tablespoon of olive oil in a large pan over low heat. Add the onions and mushrooms and cook for 10-12 minutes to soften and caramelize, stirring regularly. Clear a space for the chicken.

- Season the turkey with low sodium salt and pepper and then place it in the pan. Simmer for 15 minutes or until the chicken is cooked through. Every 5 minutes or so, spoon the sauce in the pan over the turkey.

• To assemble, divide the tomatoes between two plates. Place one turkey breast on each and then spoon the onions, mushrooms, and pan drippings over the turkey. Garnish with parsley.

STUFFED BELL PEPPERS

Ingredients:
- 5 large bell peppers
- 1 tbsp coconut oil
- 1/2 large onion, diced
- 1 tsp dried oregano
- 1/2 tsp low sodium salt
- 1 lb. ground turkey
- 1 large zucchini, halved and diced
- 3 tbsp tomato paste
- Freshly ground black pepper, to taste
- Fresh parsley, for serving

Instructions:

• Preheat the oven to 350 degrees F. Coat a small baking dish with coconut oil spray. Bring a large pot of water to a boil. Cut the stems and very top of the peppers off, removing the seeds.

• Place in boiling water for 4-5 minutes. Remove from the water and drain face-down on a paper towel.

• Heat the coconut oil in a large nonstick pan over medium heat. Add in the onion. Saute for 3-4 minutes until the onion begins to soften. Stir in the ground turkey, oregano, low sodium salt, and pepper and cook until the turkey is browned.

- Add the zucchini to the skillet as the turkey is finished cooking. Cook everything together until the zucchini is soft, and then drain any juices from the pan.

- Remove the pan from heat and stir in the tomato paste. Bake for 15 minutes.

CHILI-GARLIC OSTRICH SKEWERS

Ingredients:
- 2 Ostrich , diced
- 1 tbs. Olive Oil
- 1 tsp. Red Chilies, seeds removed & finely chopped
- 4 Garlic Cloves, minced
- 6 tbsp. fresh lemon juice

Instructions:

- Preheat the oven to 350 F or preheat the barbecue grill on high heat.

- To make sauce, combine the oil, chilies, garlic, and lemon juice in a small bowl. Set aside for a few minutes.

- Thread diced meat onto skewers and place on an oven tray lined with baking paper. Pour chili and garlic sauce over the chicken, coating well.

- Bake in the oven for 30-40 minutes or until chicken is cooked. If cooking on a grill, cook chicken for 5-6 minutes on each side.

CREAMY CHICKEN CASSEROLE

Ingredients:
- 2 cups cubed cooked chicken
- 1/2 cups cooked butternut squash
- 1/2 cup coconut cream,
- 1/4 cup coconut oil, melted
- heaping cup green peas, fresh or frozen
- 1 tbsp apple cider vinegar
- 1/2 tsp low sodium salt
- 1/2 tsp oregano
- 1/2 tsp thyme
- 1 tbsp fresh parsley

Instructions:
- In a large bowl, mash the butternut squash. Stir in the coconut cream, oil, vinegar, low sodium salt, oregano, and thyme.

- Once everything is combined, add in chicken and peas. Place the mixture into a large saucepan and cook over medium heat for 5- 8 minutes.

- Top with fresh parsley and serve warm.

SPECTACULAR SPAGHETTI AND DELISH TURKEY BALLS

Ingredients:
- 1 spaghetti squash

- Extra virgin olive oil,
- low sodium salt and pepper
- 1 tsp dried or fresh oregano

For the sauce:
- 1 lb ground turkey
- 1 small onion, chopped
- cloves garlic, minced
- 1 tbsp coconut oil
- 1 tomato, chopped
- 1/2 jar of tomato sauce
- 1 tbsp Italian seasoning
- low sodium salt and pepper to taste
- Fresh basil

Instructions:

- Preheat the oven to 400 degrees F. Using a sharp knife, cut the squash in half lengthwise. Scoop out the seeds and discard.

- Place the halves with the cut side up on a rimmed baking sheet. Drizzle with olive oil and season with low sodium salt, pepper, and oregano. Roast the squash in the oven for 40-45 minutes, until you can poke the squash .

- Let it cool until you can handle it safely. Then scrape the insides with a fork to shred the squash into strands.

- While the spaghetti squash is roasting, melt

coconut oil in a large skillet over medium heat.

- Add chopped onion and garlic and cook for 4-5 minutes. Add ground turkey and brown the meat, stirring occasionally. Season with low sodium salt and pepper.

- Add the chopped tomato, tomato sauce, and Italian seasoning and stir to combine. Simmer on low heat, stirring occasionally, while the spaghetti squash finishes roasting. Serve over spaghetti squash with basil for garnish.

COURGETTE PASTA AND TURKEY BOLOGNESE

Ingredients:
- 4 medium zucchini

For the sauce:
- 1 lb ground turkey
- 1 small onion, chopped
- 4 cloves garlic, minced
- 1 tbsp coconut oil
- 1 tomato, chopped
- 1/2 jar of tomato sauce
- 1 tbsp Italian seasoning
- salt and pepper to taste
- Fresh basil, for garnish

Instructions:

- Use a julienne peeler to slice the zucchini into noodles, stopping when you reach the seeds. Set aside.

- If cooking zucchini noodles, simply add to a skillet and saute over medium heat for 4-5 minutes.

- Melt coconut oil in a large skillet over medium heat. Add chopped onion and garlic and cook for 4-5 minutes.

- Add ground turkey and brown the meat, stirring occasionally. Season with low sodium salt and pepper.

- Add the chopped tomato, tomato sauce, and

Italian seasoning and stir to combine. Simmer on low heat, stirring occasionally.
- Add the sauce to the noodles and serve.

COURGETTE TOMATO SALAD

Ingredients:
- 2 medium zucchini
- 2 tomatoes
- cooking spray
- salt
- freshly ground black pepper
- a few sprigs fresh parsley

Instructions:
- Heat your grill to high flame. Wash zucchini and trim off the ends. Using a mandolin or vegetable peeler slice the zucchini lengthwise in thin slices.

- Lightly spray with cooking spray and season with low sodium salt and pepper, to taste. Grill the zucchini ribbons on 1 side, until lightly marked and wilted, about 1 to 2 minutes. Remove and put on a platter and let cool slightly.

- Cut up tomatoes in large chunks, season with low sodium salt and pepper to taste. Arrange on a platter with zucchini and garnish with parsley sprigs.

BRUSSELS SPROUTS

Ingredients:

- 6 oz Brussels sprouts, washed
- tbsp olive oil
- juice of 1 large lemon
- salt and fresh cracked pepper, to taste

Instructions:

- With a large sharp knife, trim off the stems, cut the brussels in half lengthwise, then place cut side down on the board and finely shred the sprouts.

- Place in a large bowl and toss with olive oil, lemon juice, salt and pepper to taste.

BEET SALAD

Ingredients:

- 2 large beets, washed and stems cut off

- 1 cup carrots, peeled and cooked
- 1 tbsp cilantro, chopped
- 1 tbsp diced onion
- 2 tbsp paleo mayonnaise
- salt and pepper

Instructions:

- Boil beets in water until soft, about 50 minutes.

- Peel and cut into small 1/2" cubes. Cook carrots until tender and cut into bite size cubes.

- Combine diced onion, carrots, beets, mayonnaise, cilantro, low sodium salt and pepper.

SASHIMI DIVINE WITH VINAIGRETTE

Ingredients:

- 2 oz sashimi tuna
- 1 tsp extra virgin olive oil
- 1 tsp fresh lemon juice
- 2 cups baby arugula
- 1 tsp capers
- salt and fresh pepper

Instructions:

- Season tuna with salt and fresh cracked pepper.

- Place arugula and capers on a plate. Combine oil and lemon juice, salt and pepper.

- Heat your grill to high heat .When the grill is hot, spray a grate with oil to prevent sticking then place tuna on the grill; cook 1 minute without moving. Flip and cook for an additional minute; remove from heat and set aside on a plate.

- Slice tuna on the diagonal and place on top of salad. Top with lemon vinaigrette and eat immediately.

GRILLED SHRIMP FENNEL SALAD

Ingredients:
- 1 lb jumbo shrimp, peeled and deveined
- 4 cups fresh arugula or baby greens
- 2 fennel bulb, thinly sliced
- 1 medium-size ripe avocado, thinly sliced

For the vinaigrette:
- 1 tbsp fresh lemon juice
- 1 tbsp extra-virgin olive oil
- 1 tbsp minced shallots
- Salt & pepper to taste

Instructions:

- Combine the lemon juice, olive oil, shallots, low sodium salt and pepper in a container with a tight-fitting lid and shake it vigorously to combine.

- Reserve cup of the vinaigrette for dressing the salad and pour the remaining vinaigrette into a medium nonreactive bowl. Put the shrimp in the bowl, season with low sodium salt and pepper and toss; let it sit for about 30 minutes.

- Prepare your outdoor grill, or heat a grill pan over medium-high heat. Grill the shrimp until just cooked through and opaque, about 1 1/2 minutes per side. Transfer to a plate.

- Divide the baby greens on four plates, top with sliced fennel, oranges, avocados and shrimp.

Season with salt and pepper to taste and drizzle with the remaining vinaigrette, about 2 tbsp per salad.

CHICKEN DELISH SALAD

Ingredients:

- 1 lb skinless boneless chicken breast, cut into 1 inch cubes

For the marinade:

- 1 tbsp lemon juice
- 1 tsp dried oregano
- 1 tsp garlic, crushed
- salt to taste
- fresh ground black pepper to taste

For the salad:

- 1 1/4 cups cucumber, peeled
- 1/4 cups diced tomato
- 1/4 cup diced bell pepper
- 1 tbsp red onion, diced
- 1/2 tsp fresh lemon juice
- 1 tsp olive oil
- 1/8 tsp dried oregano
- 1 tsp parsley
- 1/2 tsp vinegar
- salt and black pepper to taste
- 2 cups shredded lettuce
- lemon wedges for serving

Instructions:

- Marinate the chicken for at least 2-3 hours or overnight. If using wooden skewers, soak in water for at least 30 minutes if grilling outdoors.

- Combine the first 11 salad ingredients and set aside in the refrigerator to let the flavors set.

- Thread chicken on 4 skewers and cook on a hot grill (indoor or outdoor grill) until chicken is cooked though, about 10-12 minutes. Divide lettuce between four plates, top with tomato-cucumber salad, and grilled chicken. Serve with lemon wedges.

OSTRICH STEAK WITH ROASTED TOMATOES

Ingredients:

For the tomatoes:
- 2 pints cherry tomatoes, halved
- 1 tbsp extra virgin olive oil
- Stevia to taste
- salt and freshly ground pepper

For the cauliflower rice:
- 1/2 head of cauliflower, chopped coarsely

- 1/2 small onion, finely diced
- 1 tbsp coconut oil
- 1 tbsp fresh parsley, chopped
- salt and freshly ground pepper, to taste

For the meat:
- Ostrich or venison steaks
- 1 Extra virgin olive oil
- salt and freshly ground pepper
- Coconut oil, for the pan

For the sauce:
- 1/4 cup red onion, finely diced
- 1/4 cup apple cider vinegar
- 1 cup low sodium chicken stock
- 1 tbsp whole grain mustard
- salt and freshly ground pepper, to taste

Instructions:

- Preheat the oven to 400 degrees F. Place the tomatoes on a baking sheet and drizzle with olive oil and honey. Sprinkle with low sodium salt and pepper and toss to coat evenly. Bake for 15-20 minutes until soft.

- While the tomatoes are roasting, prepare the cauliflower rice. Place the cauliflower into a food processor and pulse until reduced to the size of rice grains.

- Melt the coconut oil in a nonstick skillet

over medium heat. Add the onion and cook for 5-6 minutes until translucent. Stir in the cauliflower, season with low sodium salt and pepper, and cover. Cook for 7-10 minutes until the cauliflower has softened, and then toss with parsley.

- To make the lamb, preheat the oven to 325 degrees F. Pat the ostrich or venison dry and rub with olive oil. Generously season both sides with low sodium salt and pepper.

- Heat one tablespoon of coconut oil in a cast iron skillet. When the pan is hot, add to the pan and sear for 2-3 minutes on all sides until golden brown.

- Place the skillet in the oven and bake for 5-8 minutes until the ostrich or venison reaches desired doneness. Let rest for 10 minutes before serving. While the meat is resting, add the red onion to the skillet with the pan drippings from the lamb. Saute for 3-4 minutes, then add the white wine vinegar.

- Turn the heat to high and cook until the vinegar has mostly evaporated. Add the stock and bring to a boil, cooking until the sauce reduces by half.

- Stir in the mustard, and season to taste with low sodium salt and pepper. Pour over ostrich or venison to serve.

TANTALIZING TURKEY PEPPER STIR-FRY

Ingredients:

- 2 bell peppers, sliced
- 1 cup broccoli florets
- 2 cooked and shredded turkey breasts
- 1/4 tsp chili powder
- salt and pepper to taste
- 1 tbsp coconut oil for frying

Instructions:

- Add 1 tablespoon coconut oil into a frying pan on medium heat.

- Place the sliced bell peppers into the frying pan.

- After the bell peppers soften, add in the cooked turkey meat.

- Add in the chili powder, low sodium salt and pepper.

- Mix well and stir-fry for a few more minutes.

CHEEKY CHICKEN STIR FRY

Ingredients:
- 1 lb boneless, skinless chicken breast
- 2 tbsp coconut oil
- 1 cup onion, finely chopped
- 4 cups broccoli, sliced into 3-inch spears
- 2 medium carrots, sliced
- 2 heads baby bok choy, sliced crosswise into 1-inch strips
- 1 cup shiitake mushrooms, stemmed and thinly sliced
- 1 cup zucchini, sliced
- 1 teaspoon salt
- Garlic powder to taste
- 2 cups water

Instructions:
- Rinse the chicken and pat dry. Cut into 1-inch cubes and transfer to a plate.

- Heat the coconut oil in a large skillet over medium heat Saute the onion for 8 to 10 minutes, until soft and translucent

- Add the broccoli, carrots, and chicken and saute for 10 minutes until almost tender

- Add the bok choy, mushrooms, zucchini, and low sodium salt and saute for 2 minutes

- Add 1 cup of the water, cover the skillet,

and cook for about 10 minutes, until the vegetables are wilted

- In a small bowl, dissolve the arrowroot powder in the remaining cup of water, stirring until thoroughly combined
- Season at the end with garlic powder, salt and some chili powder

TURKEY THAI BASIL

Ingredients:

- 2 lbs leftover cooked turkey, cubed or shredded
- 1 Tbsp fish sauce
- 1 Tbsp coconut aminos
- 1 Tbsp water
- Stevia to taste
- 1 tsp salt
- 1/2 tsp ground white pepper
- 1 Tbsp coconut oil
- baby bok choy, leaves pulled apart, hearts halved
- 1 red bell pepper, sliced
- 1 yellow bell pepper, sliced
- 1 large onion, sliced
- 2 cloves garlic, minced
- 1/2 cup lightly packed Thai basil leaves

Instructions:

- In a medium bowl, combine turkey with fish sauce, water, low sodium salt and pepper; stir until turkey is thoroughly coated and set aside

- Melt coconut oil in large wok or frying pan over medium-high heat

- Add bok choy, peppers, onion and garlic and saute until softened, about 8 minutes, stirring frequently

- Add contents of set-aside bowl (with the meat) to pan and stir for about 3 minutes until turkey is fully incorporated and heated through

- Remove from heat and add Thai basil, stirring until basil wilts

CHICKEN FENNEL STIR-FRY

Ingredients:
- 3 chicken breasts or the meat from 1 whole roasted chicken
- 2 tbsp coconut oil
- 1 onion
- 1 bulb of fennel
- 1 tsp each of salt, pepper, garlic powder and basil

Instructions:
- Cut the chicken into bite sized pieces. If chicken is raw, heat butter/coconut oil in a large

skillet or wok until melted.

- Add chicken and cook on medium/high heat until chicken is cooked through. (If chicken is pre-cooked, cook the vegetables first then add chicken)

- While cooking, cut the onion into bite sized pieces (1/2 inch) and thinly slice the fennel bulb into thin slivers.

- Add all to the skillet or wok, add spices and continue sauteing until all are cooked through and fragrant.

MOROCCAN MADNESS

Ingredients:
- 1 chicken breast, chopped into pieces
- 1/2 tbsp olive oil
- 1/2 onion, chopped
- 1 bell pepper, chopped
- 1 cup diced courgette
- 2 cloves garlic, minced
- 1 tsp ginger, minced
- 1 tsp cumin
- 1 tsp turmeric
- 1/2 tsp paprika
- 1/2 tbsp oregano

- 1/2 can diced tomatoes
- 1/2 cup low sodium chicken stock
- salt and pepper

Instructions:

- In a pan cook the chicken in the olive oil .Once it's finished cooking, remove from the pan and set aside.
- Add to the pan the bell pepper, onion, courgette, garlic, ginger and all spices, saute until bell pepper and onion become soft .
- Add back in the chicken along with the diced tomatoes and chicken stock, let simmer for 1o minutes.

GOLDEN GLAZED DRUMSTICKS

Ingredients:

- 8 medium chicken drumsticks, skin removed
- olive oil spray 1 cup water
- 1/3 cup rice vinegar
- 1/3 cup low sodium gluten free soy sauce
- 3 drops stevia
- 2 cloves garlic, crushed
- 1 tsp ginger, grated

- 1 tbsp chives or scallions, chopped
- 1 tsp sesame seeds

Instructions:

- In a heavy large saucepan, brown chicken on high for 3-4 minutes with a little spray oil. Add water, vinegar, soy sauce, stevia, garlic, ginger and cook on high until liquid comes to a boil.

- Reduce heat to low and simmer, covered for about 20 minutes.

- Remove cover and bring heat to high, allowing sauce to reduce down, about 8-10 minutes, until it becomes thick, turning chicken occasionally. (Keep an eye on the glaze, you don't want it to burn when it starts becoming thick) Transfer chicken to a platter and pour sauce on top.

- Top with chives and sesame seeds and serve.

SPICY GRILLED TURKEY RECIPE

Ingredients:
- thin turkey filets (3 oz each)

For the Marinade:
- 2 tbsp lemon juice
- 2 tbsp toasted sesame seeds
- 2 cloves garlic, minced
- 2 tsp fresh ginger, peeled and minced
- 2 green onions, minced
- 1/4 cup low sodium soy sauce
- Stevia to taste
- 2 tsp sesame oil

Instructions:
- Combine all marinade ingredients in a small bowl. Pour the mixture over the turkey, turn the pieces to coat evenly, cover and place in the refrigerator a minimum of three hours, but preferably overnight.
- Preheat the grill too high. Grill one side first until well browned charred, about 5 minutes, turn and cook on the second side about 3 more minutes.

SPICY PEANUT CHICKEN

Ingredients:
- 3/4 cup green onion, chopped
- 1/4 cups shredded carrots
- 1 1/4 cups cup shredded broccoli slaw
- 1 cup bean bean sprouts
- 1 tbsp chopped salt free peanuts
- lime, sliced
- cilantro for garnish (optional)

For the Peanut Sauce:
- 14.5 oz fat free chicken broth
- 1 tbsp peanut butter
- Stevia to taste
- 1 tbsp soy sauce
- 1 tbsp freshly grated ginger
- 2 cloves garlic, minced

For the chicken:
- 16 oz chicken breast, cut into thin strips
- salt and pepper
- 1 tsp chili flakes
- juice of 1/2 lime
- cloves garlic, crushed
- 1 tbsp fresh ginger, grated
- 1 tbsp soy sauce
- 1/2 tbsp sesame oilInstructions:
-     For the peanut sauce: Combine 1 cup chicken broth, peanut butter, stevia, 2 tbsp soy sauce, ginger, and 3 cloves crushed garlic in a

small saucepan and simmer over medium-low heat stirring occasionally until sauce becomes smooth and well blended, about 5-10 minutes.

- Set aside.Season chicken with low sodium salt and pepper, chili, lime, garlic, ginger and soy sauce.

- Heat a large skillet or wok until hot. Add oil and saute chicken on high heat until cooked through, about 2-3 minutes; remove from heat and set aside.

- Add 2 cloves crushed garlic,scallions,carrots, broccoli slaw and/or bean sprouts and low sodium salt, saute until tender crisp, about 1-2 minutes.

- Divide chicken between 6 bowls, top with sauteed vegetables, bean sprouts, chopped peanuts ,and garnish with cilantro and lime wedges.

CHEEKY CHICKEN SALAD

Ingredients:
- olive oil spray
- 1 tsp olive oil
- 16 oz (2 large) skinless boneless chicken breasts, cut into chunks
- Salt & pepper to taste
- 2 cups shredded romaine
- 1 cup shredded red cabbage

For the Skinny Cheeky Sauce:
- 1/2 tbsp paleo mayonnaise
- 1 tbsp scallions, chopped
- 1 1/2 tsp chili flakes

Instructions:
- Preheat the oven to 425°F. Spray a baking sheet with olive oil spray.

- Season chicken with low sodium salt and pepper, olive oil and mix well so the olive oil evenly coats all of the chicken.

- Meanwhile combine the sauce in a medium bowl. When the chicken is ready, drizzle it over the top and enjoy!

MELTING MUSTARD CHICKEN

Ingredients:
- 8 small chicken thighs, skin removed
- 1 tsp mustard powder
- 1 tbsp paleo mayonnaise
- 1 clove garlic, crushed
- 1 lime, squeezed, and lime zest
- 3/4 tsp pepper
- Salt to taste
- dried parsley

Instructions:
- Preheat the oven to 400°F. Rinse the chicken

and remove the skin and all fat. Pat dry ...place in a large bowl and season generously with low sodium salt. In a small bowl combine mustard, mayonnaise, lime juice, lime zest, garlic and pepper. Mix well. Pour over chicken, tossing well to coat.

- Spray a large baking pan with a little Pam to prevent sticking since all the fat and skin was removed from the chicken. Place chicken to fit in a single layer.

- Top the chicken with dried parsley. Bake until cooked through, about 30- 35 minutes.

- Finish the chicken under the broiler until it is golden brown. Serve chicken with the pan juices drizzled over the top.

TANTALIZING TURKEY WITH ROASTED VEGETABLES

Ingredients:
- 20 oz Turkey Breasts
- 20 medium asparagus, ends trimmed, cut in half
- 2 red bell peppers
- 1 cup carrots, sliced in half long way
- 1/4 cup extra virgin olive oil
- 1 tsp stevia
- salt and pepper to taste
- 1 tbsp fresh rosemary
- 2 cloves garlic, smashed and sliced

- 2 tbsp oregano or thyme
- 1 tbsp chopped fresh sage

Instructions:

- Preheat the oven to 425°F. Wash and dry the chicken well with a paper towel.

- Combine all the ingredients together and using your hands and arrange in a very large roasting pan.

- The vegetables should not touch the turkey or it will steam instead of roast. All ingredients should be spread out in a single layer. Bake for 35 - 40 minutes.

GRILLED OSTRICH STEAK

Ingredients:
- 2 medium ostrich steaks
- 1 tbsp vinegar
- garlic powder to taste
- black pepper to taste
- oregano
- 2 tbsp olive oil

Instructions:
- Season ostrich with vinegar and olive oil.
- Add garlic powder, oregano and mix well, let marinate at least 20 minutes.
- Broil or grill on low until the ostrich is cooked through, careful not to burn.

- Enjoy with green salad.

LEMONY CHICKEN AND ASPARAGUS

Ingredients:
- 1 1/2 pounds skinless chicken breast, cut into cubes
- salt, to taste
- 1/2 cup reduced-sodium chicken broth
- 2 tbsp reduced-sodium soy sauce
- 2 tbsp water
- 1 tbsp olive oil, divided
- 1 bunch asparagus, trimmed, cut into 2-inch pieces
- 2 cloves garlic, chopped
- 1 tbsp fresh ginger
- 2 tbsp fresh lemon juice
- fresh black pepper, to taste

Instructions:
- Lightly season the chicken with low sodium salt. In a small bowl, combine chicken broth and soy sauce. In a second small bowl combine the cornstarch and water and mix well to combine.

- Heat a large non-stick wok over medium-high heat, when hot add 1 teaspoon of the oil, then add the asparagus and cook until tender-crisp, about 3 to 4 minutes. Add the garlic and ginger and cook until golden, about 1 minute. Set aside.

- Increase the heat to high, then add 1 teaspoon

of oil and half of the chicken and cook until browned and cooked through, about 4 minutes on each side. Remove and set aside and repeat with the remaining oil and chicken. Set aside.

- Add the soy sauce mixture; bring to a boil and cook for about 1-1/2 minutes. Add lemon juice and stir well, when it simmers return the chicken and asparagus to the wok and mix well, remove from heat and serve.

DELISH CHICKEN SOUP

Ingredients:
- 5 cups reduced sodium chicken broth
- 3 cups shredded chicken breast
- 1 tomato, diced
- 2 cloves garlic, minced
- 1-1/2 cups scallions, chopped fine
- 1/3 cup cilantro, chopped fine
- lime wedges
- 2 tsp olive oil
- salt and pepper to taste
- pinch cumin
- pinch chili powder (optional)

Instructions:
- In a large pot, heat oil over medium heat. Add 1 cup of scallions and garlic. Saute about 2 minutes then add tomatoes and saute another minute, until soft.

- Add chicken stock, cumin and chili powder and bring to a boil. Simmer, covered on low for about 15-20 minutes.

- Ladle 1 cup chicken broth over the chicken and serve with a lime wedge.

CHICKEN PAPRIKA SURPRISE

Ingredients:
- 1 lb iced paprika - use all 4 colors
- 12 oz boneless skinless chicken thighs, all fat trimmed
- 8 cups water
- 1 tbsp low salt chicken Bouillon
- 1 small onion
- 2 scallions
- 1/4 cup chopped cilantro
- 2 cloves garlic
- 1 medium ripe tomato
- 1 tsp garlic powder
- 1 tsp cumin
- 1/4 tsp oregano
- 1/4 tsp ground Spanish paprika
- salt, to taste

Instructions:

- In a large pot combine paprikas, chicken,

water and chicken bouillon. Bring to a boil, covered over medium-low heat until chicken is cooked, about 20 minutes. Remove the chicken and shred, return to the pot.

- Meanwhile, in a chopper or by hand, mince the onions, scallions, cilantro, garlic, and tomato. Add to the lentils with garlic powder, cumin, oregano and cook, covered until the lentils are soft, about 25 more minutes, adding more water as needed if too thick. Adjust low sodium salt to taste as needed.

CHICKEN HEALING SOUP

Ingredients:
- 1 tsp olive oil
- 1 cup chopped carrots
- 1/2 cup chopped onions
- 1/2 cup chopped celery
- 2 cloves garlic, chopped
- 1-1/2 lbs skinless bone-in chicken breast
- 6 cups reduced sodium chicken broth
- 1/4 cup chopped parsley
- 2 bay leaves
- black pepper, to taste

Instructions:
- Heat a large heavy pot on medium heat. Add the oil, carrots, onion, celery and garlic to the pot and stir.

- Add chicken, broth, parsley, and bay leaves and bring to a boil. When boiling, reduce heat to low and cover.

- Simmer over low heat until the chicken and vegetables are tender, about 30 minutes.

- Remove the chicken, shred or cut the meat, discard the bones and return the chicken to the pot, adjust the salt if needed and add pepper.

- Simmer for 20 minutes. Discard the bay leaves and serve.

BAKED CHICKEN

Ingredients:
- 1 lb medium bone-in skinless drumsticks
- 1 tsp salt
- 1/2 tsp garlic powder
- 1/2 tsp paprika
- 1/2 tsp fresh black pepper
- 1/2 tsp cayenne pepper
- 1 tbsp paleo mayonnaise
- 1 tsp mustard powder
- Oil spray
- 1/2 cup cereal
- 2 tsp almond flour

Instructions:
- Preheat the oven to 400°F. Line a baking sheet with foil and set a rack above. Spray rack with oil.

- Crush cereal in a food processor. In a bowl mix almond flour with salt, paprika, garlic powder, black pepper and cayenne pepper. Place in a shallow dish or zip lock bag.

- Combine mayonnaise and mustard. Using a cooking brush, brush onto chicken then coat chicken with crushed cereal mixture. Place chicken on a wire rack and spray with oil. Bake for 35-40 minutes.

SOUTH AMERICAN CHICKEN

Ingredients:

- 1 whole chicken
- 1/4 cup white vinegar
- lime, juice of
- 1/2 tsp cumin
- 1 tsp garlic powder
- 1 tsp dried oregano
- Salt to taste
- 1 tsp paprika

Sauce:

- 2-3 jalapenos, seeded
- 1 tbsp fresh cilantro
- 1 tbsp olive oil
- 1 clove garlic
- 1 tbsp white vinegar
- pinch cumin
- salt and pepper to taste
- 1 tbsp coconut cream

Instructions:

- Wash chicken and remove all fat. Place in a large bowl and season generously with beer, vinegar, lime juice, low sodium salt, garlic powder, cumin and oregano. Place in a large bag and marinate overnight.

- Remove chicken from bag, cut chicken in half and place both halves on a large oven safe baking dish, skin side up.

- Discard marinade. Sprinkle chicken with paprika and a little more garlic powder and salt and bake at 425° for about 50 minutes, basting with the pan juices half way through.

ROSEMARY CHICKEN

Ingredients:
- (3 lb) chicken, washed and dried, fat removed
- 1/2 onion, chopped in large chunks
- 2 cloves garlic, smashed
- 1/2 lemon
- 2-3 sprigs rosemary
- 1 tbsp dried rosemary
- salt and pepper to taste

Instructions:

- Heat oven to 425°F. Season chicken inside and out with salt, pepper, and rosemary. Squeeze lemon juice on the outside of the chicken and stuff the remains of the lemon along with onion, garlic, rosemary sprigs inside the chicken.

- Roast the chicken until the internal temperature is 165°F, about 50-60 minutes (Insert thermometer between the leg and the thigh). Let the bird rest for 10 minutes before carving.

- Serve with steamed vegetables of choice

SESAME TURKEY

Ingredients:

- 18 oz turkey breasts
- salt and pepper to taste
- 1 tsp sesame oil
- 2 tsp low sodium soy sauce gluten free
- 1 tbsp toasted sesame seeds
- 1/2 tsp salt
- 2 tsp olive oil

Instructions:

- Preheat the oven to 425°. Spray a baking sheet with non-stick oil spray.
- Combine the sesame oil and soy sauce in a bowl, and the sesame seeds and salt.
- Place turkey in the bowl with the oil and soy sauce, then into the sesame seed mixture to coat well. Place on the baking sheet; lightly spray the top of the chicken with oil spray and bake for 8 - 10 minutes.
- Turn over and cook another 4 - 5 minutes longer or until cooked through.
- Serve with cauliflower rice or fried celeriac

VINEGAR CHICKEN

Ingredients:

- 1 cup chicken broth
- 8 lean chicken thighs, skin removed
- Stevia to taste
- Salt & pepper to taste

- 1/2 cup red wine vinegar
- 1 tbsp tomato paste
- 1 tsp butter
- 3/4 cup shallot, thinly sliced
- 2 cloves garlic, thinly sliced
- 1/2 cup dry white wine
- 2 tbsp coconut cream
- 2 tbsp fresh chopped parsley

Instructions:

- Season chicken with salt and pepper.
- In a medium saucepan, combine vinegar, stevia, 3/4 cup chicken broth and tomato paste. Boil for about 5 minutes, until it reduces down to about 3/4 cup. Remove from heat.
- In a large skillet, melt butter over medium-low heat and add chicken. Cook on both sides, until brown, about 6-8 minutes.
- Remove chicken and set aside. Add the shallots and garlic to the skillet and cook on low until soft, about 5 minutes.
- Pour the sauce over the chicken, add the wine, remaining broth, low sodium salt and pepper. Cover and simmer for about 20 minutes until tender.
- Remove the chicken, add cream and stir into the sauce (if sauce dries up, add more broth). Boil for a few minutes then return chicken to the skillet. Top with fresh parsley.

CHICKEN DELISH

Ingredients:
- 1/2 tbsp olive oil
- 1 large chicken breast halves, bone in, skin removed
- salt and pepper to taste
- 1/2 medium head of cauliflower, cut into florets
- 1 medium onion, sliced thinly
- 2 cloves of garlic, sliced thinly
- 1 dried chili pepper, sliced
- 1/3 cup dry white wine
- 1 cup reduced sodium chicken stock
- 1 sprig rosemary

Instructions:
- Preheat the oven to 375°F. Cut chicken in half to make 4 pieces, leaving the bone on.

- Heat oil in a large, oven safe saute pan with straight sides over medium- high heat. Season the chicken with low sodium salt and pepper and brown 2-3 minutes per side. Remove chicken and set aside.

- Reduce heat to medium and add onion, cauliflower florets, garlic and chill.Saute, stirring frequently, for 2-3 minutes until vegetables start to brown.

- Add the white wine, cherry peppers and

additional optional liquid. Raise heat and allow to boil for about 2 minutes before adding chicken stock. Add chicken breasts back into the pan, bone side down, sprinkle rosemary on top, bring to a boil and then place the pan in the oven, uncovered.

- Cook for 20-25 minutes or until chicken reaches 165°F. Remove from oven carefully, with towel or kitchen gloves, serve and enjoy!

COURGETTE SPAGHETTI WITH CHICKEN

Ingredients:
- 2 skinless chicken breast halves, diced
- cooking spray
- 1/2 tsp each of dried oregano and dried basil
- salt and pepper to taste
- 2 courgettes spiralized
- 2 cups grape tomatoes, halved
- 6 cloves garlic, smashed and coarsely chopped
- 1 tsp extra virgin olive oil
- 4 tbsp chopped fresh basil

Instructions:
- Season chicken generously with salt, pepper, oregano and basil.

- Heat a large skillet on high heat. When hot, spray with oil and courgette pasta and cook for 3 minutes. Set aside.

- Add olive oil and chicken to the same skillet. Cook for about 3-4 minutes, until it is no longer pink. Remove chicken and set aside.

- Add olive oil to the skillet on high heat. Add garlic and saute until golden brown.

- Add tomatoes, salt and pepper and reduce heat to medium-low. Saute about 4-5 minutes.

- Add courgettes pasta, fresh basil and chicken to tomatoes and toss well.

CHICKEN PEA STIR FRY

Ingredients:

For the sauce:
- 1 tbsp low sodium soy sauce
- 1 tbsp fresh lime juice
- 1 tbsp water

For the Stir Fry:
- 1 lb skinless, boneless chicken breast, sliced thin
- salt, to taste
- 1 tbsp sesame oil
- 1 tsp fresh garlic, minced
- 1 tsp fresh ginger, grated
- 2 cups sugar snap peas

- 1 cup carrots, sliced diagonally
- scallions for garnish

Instructions:

- Combine soy sauce, lime juice, water in a small bowl, mix together and set aside.

- Season chicken lightly with low sodium salt. Heat a large wok over high heat. When the wok is very hot, add half of the oil, then add the chicken.

- Stir fry, stirring occasionally until the chicken is cooked through and browned, about 3-4 minutes. With a slotted spoon, remove the chicken and set aside. Reduce heat to medium.

- Add the remaining oil to the wok; add the garlic and ginger, stir for 20 seconds. Add the sugar snap peas and carrots, stirring over medium high heat until tender crisp, about 3-4 minutes.

- Return the chicken to the wok, add the soy sauce-lime mixture, mix well and cook another 30 seconds to one minute. Serve immediately and top with fresh scallions.

SCRUMPTIOUS COD IN DELISH SAUCE

Ingredients:

- 1 lb cod filets
- 1/3 cup almond flour
- 1/2 tsp low sodium salt

- 2-3 tbsp extra virgin olive oil
- 1 tbsp walnut oil, divided
- 3/4 cup low sodium chicken stock
- 1 tbsp lemon juice
- 1/4 cup capers, drained
- 1 tbsp fresh parsley, chopped

Instructions:

- Stir the almond flour and low sodium salt together in a shallow bowl. Rinse off the fish and pat dry with a paper towel. Dredge the fish in the almond flour mixture to coat.

- Heat enough olive oil to coat the bottom of a large skillet over medium-high heat along with one tablespoon walnut oil. Working in batches, add the cod and cook for 2-3 minutes per side to brown. Remove to a plate and set aside.

- Add the chicken stock, lemon juice, and capers to the same skillet and scrape any browned bits off the bottom. Simmer to reduce the sauce by almost half. Remove from heat and stir in the remaining oil.

- To serve, divide the cod onto plates, drizzle with the sauce, and sprinkle with parsley.

BAKED DILL SALMON

Ingredients:

- 2 6-oz. salmon filets

- 2 zucchini, halved lengthwise and thinly sliced
- 1/4 red onion, thinly sliced
- 1 tsp fresh dill, chopped
- lemon slices
- 1 tbsp fresh lemon juice
- Extra virgin olive oil, for drizzling
- salt and pepper to taste

Instructions:

- Preheat the oven to 350 F. Prepare a baking tray

- Place half of the zucchini, red onion, dill, and one lemon slice. Drizzle with olive oil and sprinkle with low sodium salt and pepper.

- Place a salmon filet on top and drizzle with the lemon juice. Season with low sodium salt and pepper. Repeat with the remaining ingredients.

- Bake for 15-20 minutes until the salmon is opaque.

PRAWN GARLIC FRIED RICE

Ingredients:

- 1 tbsp coconut oil
- 1 cup white onion, finely chopped
- 2 cloves garlic, minced
- 8 oz. prawns peeled and deveined
- 1 medium carrot, chopped

- 1/2 cup peas
- 2 cups cooked cauliflower rice
- 2 eggs, beaten
- salt and pepper, to taste

Instructions:

- Heat a wok or large pan over medium-high heat. Melt the coconut oil and add the onion and garlic to the pan.

- Cook for 3-4 minutes until the onion starts to soften. Add the shrimp and cook for 1 minute.

- Add the carrot, peas, and bell pepper to the pan. Cook for 3-4 minutes, and then stir in the cauliflower rice.

- Clear a circle in the center of the pan and pour in the beaten eggs. Stir to scramble the eggs and then combine with the other ingredients.

LEMON AND THYME SUPER SALMON

Ingredients:

- 32 oz piece of salmon
- 1 sliced lemon
- 1 tsp lemon juice
- salt and pepper to taste
- 1 tbsp fresh thyme
- Olive oil, for drizzling

Instructions:

- Line a baking sheet with parchment paper and place salmon, skin side down on the dish.

- Season salmon with salt and pepper and top with sliced lemon and thyme.

- Place the baking sheet in a cold oven, then turn the heat to 400 degrees F. Bake for 25 minutes. Add lemon juice and serve immediately.

DELICIOUS SALMON IN HERB CRUST

Ingredients:
- 2 salmon filets
- 1 small onion, peeled and quartered
- 2 garlic cloves, peeled
- 1 sprig lemongrass, coarsely chopped
- A piece ginger root, peeled
- 1 red chili pepper

Instructions:

- Preheat oven to 390 F. Start by making the herb crust: combine the onion, garlic, lemongrass, ginger in the smallest bowl of a food processor

- Process into a coarse paste.

- Put the salmon filets in an oven dish and spread the herb paste on top.

- Bake for approx. 12-15 minutes until done, depending on the thickness of your filets.

- Serve with veggies of your choice and enjoy!

SALMON MUSTARD DELISH

Ingredients:
- 1/2 tsp mustard seed
- 1/2 tsp garlic powder
- 1/4 tsp salt
- 1/4 tsp black pepper
- 1/4 tsp dried dill
- 1 1/2 lb salmon

Instructions:

- Preheat the oven to 425°F. Grind the mustard seeds with a mortar and pestle until mustard seeds are cracked.

- Combine with salt, pepper, dill and garlic

powder.

- Spread the mixture over the salmon evenly, and place on a baking pan with a non-stick rack.

- Bake for 15 to 20 minutes, until the flesh flakes easily with a fork. If you prefer salmon that is medium-rare, 15 minutes should be enough.

- Enjoy!

SPICY SALMON

Ingredients:

For the Salmon:

- 6 ounce Sockeye Salmon Filets
- 1/2 teaspoon of Cinnamon
- 1 teaspoon of Coriander
- 1 teaspoon of Cumin
- 1/8 teaspoon of Ground Cloves
- 1/2 teaspoon of Cardamom
- salt to taste
- 1 Tablespoon of coconut butter

For the Lime Mustard dressing:

- 1 cup of olive oil
- 1 Tablespoon of Lime Juice
- 2 teaspoons of mustard powder
- Pinch of low sodium salt

Instructions:

- Preheat the oven to 425°F. Grind all of the spices together with a mortar and pestle until mustard seeds are cracked, most are powder, and everything is well blended.

- Spread the mixture over the salmon evenly, and place on a baking pan with a non-stick rack.

- Bake for 15 to 20 minutes, until the flesh flakes easily with a fork. If you prefer salmon that is medium-rare, 15 minutes should do the trick.

- Enjoy with your favorite sauteed greens, or mixed salad.

MOUTHWATERING STUFFED SALMON

Ingredients:

- 1 lb wild Alaskan or sockeye salmon, cut into 2 pieces
- 6 oz raw shrimp, peeled, deveined and chopped
- 1 large egg
- 1 tbsp raw onions, chopped
- 2 tbsp Italian flat leaf parsley, chopped
- 2 tbsp almond meal (or almond flour)
- 2 tbsp coconut butter
- 1 clove garlic, minced
- salt and pepper to taste

Instructions:

- Preheat the oven to 400F ; Pat dry the salmon filets with a paper towel.

- Combine the cinnamon, coriander, cumin, cloves, and cardamom. Sprinkle evenly over the salmon filet side.

- Heat an oven safe skillet to medium high heat. Add the coconut butter and let it melt.

- Place the salmon filet side down and let sear for about 1-2 minutes. Flip and sear on the skin side for 1 minute.

- Place the skillet inside the oven, with the skin side down. Bake at 400F for 6-7 minutes.

- Combine dressing, lime juice, low sodium salt, and mustard. Dip with salmon and enjoy!

GARLIC LEMON SHRIMP

Ingredients:
- 1 lb shrimp, deveined
- 3-4 cloves of garlic, chopped
- 1/2 fresh lemon juice
- 1 tbsp olive oil
- 1/8 of salt
- Fresh ground pepper (to taste)
- 1 tbsp fresh parsley, chopped for garnish

Instructions:
- Preheat the broiler, if using. Heat the olive oil in a heavy skillet over medium-low heat.

- Add the garlic and saute, stirring frequently, for about five minutes, until the garlic is softened but not browned.

- Add the shrimp, raise the heat to medium high, and sprinkle with low sodium salt, pepper, paprika, and red pepper.

- Cook for three minutes on each side or until the shrimp are completely opaque. Serve hot

COURGETTE PESTO AND SHRIMP

Ingredients:

For the Pesto Sauce:

- 1/4 cup pesto
- salt & Pepper
- 1 Small Zucchini into zoodles
- 1/2 lb Shrimp (peeled & deveined)
- 1 garlic clove minced
- 1 tsp ghee

Instructions:

- Heat pan to medium-high heat. Add ghee and garlic. Saute for about a minute.
- Add shrimp. Saute for about a minute on each side.

- Add salt, pepper and zoodles. Saute for another minute. Stir in pesto and stir well to combine.

- Remove from heat and dish onto a plate or bowl.

EASY SHRIMP STIR FRY

Ingredients:
- 1 lb of wild shrimp
- 1 tbsp Lemon juice
- 2 Cloves of garlic, minced
- 2 Tablespoons of olive oil
- Dash of red pepper flakes

Instructions:
- Heat oil in a pan. Stir in shrimp salt ,pepper and minced garlic and pepper flakes.
- Cook shrimp over medium heat for 3 minutes per side. Add lemon juice and serve.

PRAWN SALAD BOATS

Ingredients:
- 1 lb shrimp, cooked
- 1 medium tomato, diced
- 1 cucumber, peeled and diced
- tablespoons olive oil
- 1 tablespoon coconut cream
- Juice of 1 lemon
- 1/2 tsp dried dill
- 1/2 tsp celery seed
- 1/4 tsp low sodium salt
- 1/4 tsp pepper
- Endive or big lettuce leaf, for serving

Instructions:

- In a large saute pan, heat olive oil over medium heat. Add onion, beans, and saute until tender -approximately 10 minutes.

- Add garlic, lime juice, and chili powder and continue to cook for an additional 5 minutes.

- Add spinach and shrimp. Continue to cook for approximately 7-10 more minutes until spinach has wilted and shrimp is done.

- In a medium bowl, mix the coconut cream, and lemon juice until combined.
- Add the shrimp, tomato, cucumbers, capers, and spices.
- Mix until everything is incorporated. Add additional low sodium salt and pepper to taste. Serve in endive leaves.

CHEEKY CURRY SHRIMP

Ingredients:
- 1 lb raw, peeled, tail on shrimp
- 1 tsp curry powder
- 1 tsp garlic powder
- 1 tsp ground coriander
- 1/2 tsp ground ginger
- salt and black pepper to taste
- 1 tbsp olive oil

Instructions:

- Rinse shrimp under cold water and pat dry with a paper towel. Place shrimp in a large Ziploc bag.

- In a small mixing bowl, curry powder, coriander, garlic powder, ground ginger, low sodium salt, and pepper.

- Pour spice mixture over shrimp, seal bag, and toss to evenly coat.

- Place shrimp in the fridge and allow to marinate for at least an hour.

- Preheat the grill to high heat. Grill shrimp for about 6 minutes.

COURGETTE SHRIMP TOMATO

Ingredients:
- 1 pound fresh shrimp, peeled and deveined
- 4-5 medium courgettes sliced
- 1 onion, chopped
- 2 cloves garlic, chopped
- 1 can diced tomatoes, with liquid (14 oz.)
- 1/2 cup broth
- 1/2 tsp red chili flake
- 1 tsp fresh oregano
- Salt & pepper
- 1 tbsp olive oil

Instructions:

- Heat a tablespoon oil in a large skillet over medium heat and toss the onion in. Saute for 1 or 2 minutes.

- Add the courgettes and garlic and saute for 1 to 2 minutes more.

- Add tomato, chili flakes, oregano, salt & pepper, and broth and simmer for 10 minutes. Add the shrimp to the and stir to combine.

- Cook over low heat until shrimp is pink and cooked through. Adjust seasoning with salt and pepper. Enjoy!

SHRIMP WITH VEGGIE STIR FRY

Ingredients:
- 1lb shrimp
- 1 tsp. of coconut oil
- 1/2 cup of thinly sliced onion
- 1/2 red bell pepper. thinly sliced
- 1 cup of full fat coconut milk
- 1 tbsp. fish sauce
- 1 minced garlic cloves
- 1 tsp minced ginger
- 1 tbsp curry powder
- 1 tbsp. of chopped cilantro

Instructions:
- In a large bowl mix fish sauce, garlic and ginger.

- Heat the oil in a wok over medium-high heat.

Once it starts to shimmer add onion and bell pepper.

- Stir-fry the onions until they start to brown around the edges, about 2 minutes.
- Add the shrimp, coconut milk and fish sauce mixture. Cook for 10 minutes and top with cilantro and serve.

SPICY SALMON

Ingredients:
- Stevia to taste
- 1 1/2 lemons, juice of
- 1/2 tsp garlic powder
- 1 tbsp soy sauce, reduced sodium gluten free
- 14 oz wild salmon filets, cut into 4 pieces
- 1 clove crushed garlic
- 1 tbsp chili flakes
- 7 oz sliced shiitake mushrooms
- 1 tbsp fresh ginger, finely minced
- 1 cup snap peas
- 1/2 cup sliced scallions, divided
- 1 tbsp black sesame seeds

Instructions:
- Mix stevia, juice of half a lemon, garlic powder, and 1 tbsp of the soy sauce in a bowl. Add salmon to marinade and set aside in the refrigerator for up to 30 minutes turning once after 15 minutes; reserve the marinade.

- Add the remaining ingredients: 2 tbsp soy sauce, remaining lemon juice, crushed garlic, and chili flakes. Add mushrooms, ginger, snap peas, 1/4 cup scallions and cook on medium heat for 5 minutes.

- Meanwhile, heat a nonstick skillet on medium heat sprayed lightly with cooking spray, remove salmon from marinade but do not discard, cook salmon 2 minutes on each side then add the marinade, cover and cook on low heat for 5 minutes.

- Serve the vegetables in a dish and top with salmon, remaining scallions and sesame seeds.

DELISH SKEWERED SHRIMP

Ingredients:
- 1-1/2 lbs large shrimp, peeled and deveined
- Chili flakes, garlic flakes, onion powder to taste

Instructions:
- Preheat the grill. Thread shrimp on skewers and season.

- Cook shrimp over medium/hot flame. When shrimp start to turn pink. Repeat every 3 to 4 minutes until done.

OREGANO PRAWNS

Ingredients:

- 1 tbsp finely chopped fresh oregano or 1 tsp dried
- 10 tiger prawns
- 1/2 tsp salt
- 1/4 tsp fresh pepper
- 1 tsp olive oil
- 1 garlic clove, minced

Instructions:

- Preheat broiler. Line a broiling pan with aluminum foil.

- Add prawns Season with low sodium salt, pepper and oregano. Add garlic, drizzle with oil.

- Arrange filets in a single layer on the prepared pan. Broil about 8 inches from the heat until the topping is browned.

TOMATO TILAPIA

Ingredients:

- 1 tbsp extra virgin olive oil
- 6 oz tilapia filets
- 2 garlic cloves, crushed
- 2 shallots, minced
- 2 tomatoes, chopped
- 2 tbsp capers
- 1/4 cup white wine
- salt and fresh pepper

Instructions:

- Brush fish with 1 tbsp olive and season with low sodium salt and pepper.

- In a medium saute pan, heat remaining olive oil. Add garlic and shallots and saute on medium-low about 4-5 minutes. Add tomatoes and season with low sodium salt and pepper. Add wine and saute until wine reduces, about 5 minutes. Add capers and saute an additional minute.

- Meanwhile, set the broiler to low and place fish about 8 inches from the flame. Broil until the fish is cooked through, about 7 minutes.

- Place fish on a platter and top with tomato caper sauce.

PRAWN ASPARAGUS STIR FRY

Ingredients:

- 2 tbsp low sodium soy sauce
- 1 tsp sherry
- 2 tbsp grated peeled fresh ginger
- 1 tsp sesame oil
- 1 pound asparagus, trimmed and cut diagonally into 2-inch pieces
- chili pepper, sliced
- 2 cloves garlic, chopped
- 1 bell pepper, sliced

- 1 lb large tiger prawns, cleaned
- salt and pepper to taste

Instructions:

- Stir together soy sauce, sherry and ginger; set aside.

- In a wok, heat 1 tsp sesame oil over medium-high heat until hot. Add prawns and cook until white, about 3 minutes. Remove from wok and set aside.

- Add remaining oil to wok. When oil is hot, add asparagus and cook for 5 minutes or until tender-crisp, stirring frequently. Add garlic.

- Add peppers and stir for another minute. Add prawns back into the wok. Pour sauce over everything and mix for another minute.

CILANTRO FISH DELISH

Ingredients:
- 1/2 pounds fresh cod or any white fish
- 1/4 teaspoon + 1/8 teaspoon ground cumin
- salt and freshly ground black pepper
- 2 teaspoons extra-virgin olive oil
- 2 garlic cloves, crushed
- 2 tablespoons lime juice
- 3 to 4 tablespoons chopped fresh cilantro

Instructions:
- Season the fish with cumin, and low sodium salt and pepper to taste.

- Heat a large nonstick skillet over medium-high heat. Add 1 teaspoon of the oil to the pan, then add half of the fish. Cook them undisturbed for about 2 minutes. Turn the shrimp over and cook until opaque throughout, about 1 minute. Transfer to a plate.

- Add the remaining 1 teaspoon oil and the remaining fish to the pan and cook, undisturbed, for about 2 minutes. Turn the shrimp over, add the garlic, and cook until the shrimp is opaque throughout, about 1 minute. Return the first batch to the skillet, mix well so that the garlic is evenly incorporated and remove the pan from the heat.

- Squeeze the lime juice over all the shrimp. Add the cilantro, toss well, and serve with cauliflower rice

PERFECT PRAWNS

Ingredients:
- 1 tsp extra virgin olive oil
- 1 lb jumbo prawns, peeled and deveined
- 2 garlic cloves, chopped
- 1 tsp crushed red pepper flakes
- fresh pepper to taste
- 2 tablespoons of capers (rinsed)
- 1/4 cup of white wine
- 1 cup clam juice
- juice from 1 lemon
- generous handful of chopped parsley
- celeriac mash

Instructions:
- Heat olive oil in a skillet. Add garlic, pepper flakes, and saute 2-3 minutes.
- Add wine, clam juice, lemon juice, parsley, low sodium salt and pepper, and stir. Cook for another 2-3 minutes.
- Add prawns and cook for 2-3 minutes.

FISH FILET DELUXE

Ingredients:
- white fish filets, about 5 oz each
- 1 tsp olive oil
- salt and fresh pepper, to taste

- 4 sprigs fresh herbs (parsley, rosemary, oregano)
- 1 lemon, sliced thin
- 4 large pieces heavy duty aluminum foil

Instructions:

- Place the fish in the center of the foil, season with low sodium salt and pepper and drizzle with olive oil. Place a slice of lemon on top of each piece of fish, then a sprig of herbs on each. Fold up the edges so that it's completely sealed and no steam will escape, creating a loose tent.

- Heat half of the grill (on one side) on high heat with the cover closed. When the grill is hot, place the foil packets on the side of the grill with the burners off (indirect heat) and close the grill.

- Serve with green salad and paleo dressing.

GAMBAS AJILLO

Ingredients:
- lb large shrimp, peeled and deveined
- 6 cloves garlic, sliced thin
- 1 tbsp Spanish olive oil
- crushed red pepper flakes
- pinch paprika
- salt

Instructions:
- In a large skillet, heat oil on medium heat and add the garlic and red pepper flakes. Saute until golden, about 2 minutes being careful not to burn.

- Add shrimp and season with salt and paprika. Cook 2-3 minutes until shrimp is cooked through. Do not overcook or it will become tough and chewy.

PEACHY PRAWN COCONUT

Ingredients:

- 1 red bell pepper, sliced thin
- 1 tsp olive oil
- 1 lb prawn
- scallions, thinly sliced, white and green parts separated
- 1/2 cup cilantro

- 2 cloves garlic, minced
- salt (to taste)
- 1/2 tsp crushed red pepper flakes (to taste)
- 14.5 oz can diced tomatoes
- 14 oz can light coconut milk
- 1/2 lime, squeezed

Instructions:

- In a medium pot, heat oil on low. Add red peppers and saute until soft (about 4 minutes). Add scallion whites, 1/4 cup cilantro, red pepper flakes and garlic. Cook for 1 minute.

- Add tomatoes, coconut milk and low sodium salt to taste, cover and simmer on low for about 10 minutes to let the flavors blend together and to thicken the sauce.

- Add prawns and cook for 5 minutes. Add lime juice.

- To serve, divide equally among 4 bowls and top with scallions and cilantro.

- Serve with cauliflower rice

DIVINE SEAFOOD STEW

Ingredients:
- dozen little clams, scrubbed and clean
- 1 lb large shrimp, peeled and deveined
- 1 lb scallops
- 1 tbsp extra virgin olive oil
- cloves garlic, minced
- 1/2 onion, chopped
- 1 tomato, diced
- 1 tablespoon dry white wine
- 1/4 cup water
- 1 bay leaf
- 1/2 cup fresh parsley, finely chopped
- salt and fresh pepper to taste

Instructions:
- In a large heavy pot, saute garlic and onion in olive oil over medium flame for about 2 minutes. Add tomatoes, wine, bay leaf, 1/4 cup parsley, low sodium salt and pepper and simmer for 5 minutes.

- Add the clams, mix well and cover. Cook for about 5 minutes or until all the clams open (discard any closed clams).

- Add shrimp and scallops and cook for an additional 2-3 minutes, until seafood is completely cooked. Ladle into bowls and top with a little fresh parsley.

BRUSSELS MUSSELS

Ingredients:

- 1 tbsp extra virgin olive oil
- 1/4 cup minced shallot
- 1 diced carrot and celery stick
- 2 garlic cloves, thinly sliced
- 1 tsp crushed red pepper
- 1/2 cup dry white wine
- 1lbs (48 to 50) live mussels, scrubbed and debearded
- 1 tbsp chopped parsley, for garnish

Instructions:

- In a large saucepan, heat the olive oil over medium-high heat until hot. Add the shallot, garlic and crushed red pepper and cook until fragrant, about 1 minute. Add the wine and boil until reduced by half, about 3 minutes.

- Stir in the mussels, cover and cook until the mussels open, 6 to 8 minutes; discard any mussels that do not open. Season lightly with low sodium salt, then transfer the mussels and sauce to a platter. Sprinkle with chopped parsley and serve right away.

ROASTED DELISH FISH FILET

Ingredients:
- white fish filets of choice, 8 oz each
- 1 tsp olive oil
- 2 cloves garlic
- 2 tbsp fresh rosemary or fresh oregano
- Low sodium salt and fresh pepper
- fresh lemon wedges for serving

Instructions:
- Preheat the oven to 450°F. Rinse and dry fish well. Line a broiler rack with aluminum foil. Lightly spray with oil.

- Rub fish with 1 tsp olive oil and season with low sodium salt and pepper, garlic and rosemary.

- Place skin side down on the oven rack. Drizzle remaining oil and bake until the fish is cooked through, about 15-20 minutes.

- Serve with cauliflower rice

TUNA STEAK

Ingredients:
- 16 oz sushi grade tuna
- 1 tsp toasted sesame oil
- Salt & pepper to taste
- 2 cups arugula

soy-ginger vinaigrette:
- 1 tbsp minced ginger

- 1 tbsp minced green onion
- 1 tbsp minced garlic
- 1/2 cup balsamic vinegar
- 1/4 cup red wine
- 1/4 cup soy sauce
- Stevia to taste
- 1 tsp toasted sesame oil
- 1 tsp mustard powder

Instructions:

- Rub the tuna steaks with 1 tsp oil, and sprinkle with low sodium salt and pepper. Place the tuna steaks in a very hot saute pan and cook for only 1 minute on each side. Set aside on a platter.

- Meanwhile, prepare salad and soy vinaigrette. Lightly coat salad with vinaigrette. Slice tuna steaks and place on top of arugula. Drizzle additional vinaigrette over the top.

CREOLE PRAWNS

Ingredients:

- 1 tsp olive oil
- medium onion, chopped
- 1/2 cup green bell pepper, chopped
- 1/2 cup celery, chopped
- cloves of garlic, minced
- 14-ounce can of diced tomatoes
- 8 oz tomato passata
- 1/4 teaspoon of cayenne pepper
- 1/4 tsp salt free Cajun Seasoning
- 1 bay leaf
- 1 tsp almond flour
- 2 tbsp water
- 1 lb of large shrimp, peeled and deveined
- 1 medium scallion, sliced
- 1 tbsp fresh parsley, chopped
- salt to taste
- Chili flakes to taste

Instructions:

- In a large skillet, heat the olive oil over medium heat. Add the chopped onion, green bell pepper, garlic and celery and saute until tender. Add tomatoes and tomato passata, cayenne pepper, cajun spice, bay leaf and bring to a boil. Cover and reduce heat to low and simmer for 20-30 minutes.

- Make a slurry of the almond flour and water and stir into the tomato mixture. Continue cooking for another 5 minutes. Lightly season the shrimp with the Cajun seasoning and add immediately to the tomato mixture. Cook for another 5 to 6 minutes, or until shrimp is opaque and cooked through, adjust low sodium salt if needed.

- Add chopped green onion and parsley and serve with cauliflower rice

TURKEY TACO SALAD

Ingredients:

- 1/2 lbs leftover turkey, cooked and chopped
- 1 1/2 tbsp taco seasoning
- 1 tsp olive oil
- 1 tsp rice vinegar
- 1/4 cup water
- 3 cups Shredded lettuce
- Optional Toppings : sliced olives, tomatoes, red onion, avocado, bell peppers
- crushed sweet potato chips

Instructions:

- To make the taco Seasoning mix together, 4 tbsp. chili powder, 1 tsp each garlic powder, onion powder, and oregano, 2 tsp each paprika and cumin, 4 tsp salt, and 1/4 tsp red pepper flakes

- Then, in a skillet, heat the oil and add in chicken - I like to fry it for a minute to give some extra flavor. Add in water and taco seasoning, let simmer until liquid is gone.

- Meanwhile, shred, chop, and dice all your toppings. Assemble, lettuce, optional toppings, chicken, dressing, and crushed chips.

AMAZING TURKEY SALAD

Ingredients:
For the Turkey:
- 1 lb boneless turkey breasts
- 1 tbsp olive oil
- salt and pepper, to taste

For the Salsa:
- 1 large tomato, quartered
- 1/2 red onion, cut into large chunks
- 1 garlic clove, peeled
- 1 small bunch of cilantro leaves
- Juice of 1 lime
- salt and pepper, to taste

Instructions:

- Preheat the oven to 375 F. Bake turkey breasts dipped in olive oil on a baking sheet for 35 to 40 minutes, until no longer pink in the center.

- While baking, add all salsa ingredients to a food processor and pulse using the chopping blade until finely chopped. Transfer the salsa to a large bowl and clean out the food processor. You will be using it to shred the turkey.

- If you don't have a food processor, just dice the tomato, onion, pepper, cilantro and garlic and add to a bowl with the lime juice, low sodium salt and pepper.

- Remove the turkey from the oven and let it cool. Once cool enough to handle, cut each breast into three or four smaller pieces and add to the food processor. Pulse using the chopping blade until shredded.

- Add turkey to a bowl with salsa and mix well with a fork. Refrigerate for at least two hours until the turkey salad is chilled.

MACADAMIA CHICKEN SALAD

Ingredients:
- 1 lb organic chicken breast
- 1 tsp macadamia nut oil, or oil of choice
- salt and pepper to taste
- 1/2 cup macadamia nuts, chopped
- 1/2 cup diced celery
- 2 tbsp julienned basil
- 1 tablespoon olive oil
- 2 teaspoons rice vinegar
- 1 tbsp lemon juice

Instructions:
- Preheat the oven to 350 degrees. Place chicken breasts on a sheet tray, drizzle with oil and a pinch of low sodium salt and pepper.

- Bake for about 35 minutes until cooked through. Remove from the oven and let cool.

- In a large bowl shred chicken. Add nuts, celery, basil, dressing, and a pinch of low sodium salt and pepper.

ROSY CHICKEN SUPREME SALAD

Ingredients:

For the chicken:
- 1 lb chicken mince, free range of course
- 1 long red chili, finely chopped with the seeds
- 2 garlic cloves, finely chopped

- Little knob of fresh ginger, peeled and finely chopped
- 1 stem lemon grass, pale section only, finely chopped

1/2 bunch of coriander stems washed and finely chopped

- 1/2 tbsp fish sauce
- 1/2 lime rind grated
- 1/2 lime, juiced
- A pinch of salt
- Coconut oil for frying

For the salad:

- 1/4 red cabbage, thinly sliced
- large carrot, peeled and grated
- 1/2 Spanish onion, thinly sliced
- 1 tbsp green spring onion, chopped
- 1/2 bunch of fresh coriander leaves (saved from the stems used in the chicken)
- A handful of fresh mint or Thai basil if available
- 1/2 cup crushed roasted cashews or some sesame seeds

For the dressing:
- 1 tbsp olive oil
- 1 tbsp lime juice
- 1 tbsp fish sauce
- small red chili, finely chopped

Instructions:

- Heat 1 tbsp of coconut oil in a large frying pan or a wok too high. Throw in lemongrass, chili, garlic, coriander stems and ginger and stir fry for about a minute until fragrant.

- Add chicken mince and lime zest. Stir and break apart the mince with a wooden spoon until separated into small chunks.

- Add fish sauce and lime juice. Stir through and cook for a further few minutes. Total cooking time for the chicken should be about 10 minutes. Prepare the salad base by mixing together sliced red cabbage, onion grated carrot, and fresh herbs.

- Mix all dressing ingredients and toss through the salad. Serve cooked chicken mince on top of the dressed salad and topped with roasted cashews, dried shallots, coconut flakes and extra fresh herbs.

TURKEY SPROUTS SALAD

Ingredients:

- 1/2 pound of Brussels sprouts
- 1/2 cup chopped almonds
- 2 turkey breasts, chopped
- 1/2 white onion, finely diced

Vinaigrette:

- 2 tbsp Apple Cider Vinegar
- 1 tbsp quality mustard powder
- 1 tbsp avocado oil
- Stevia to taste
- salt & pepper to taste

Instructions:

- Cut the Brussels sprouts in half and thinly slice. Chop the half cup of almonds. Finely dice the white onion.

- Remove the breasts and chop into bite-sized pieces. Combine all of these ingredients into a large bowl and gently toss the Brussels sprouts salad.

- Whipping up the vinaigrette takes seconds. Add all ingredients to a small bowl and whisk until smooth. Pour over the Brussels sprouts salad and toss to bring together.

BASIL AVOCADO BONANZA SALAD

Ingredients:
- 2 boneless, skinless chicken or turkey breasts (cooked and shredded)
- 1/2 cup fresh basil leaves, stems removed
- 1 large ripe avocado, pit and skin removed
- 2 tbsp. extra virgin olive oil
- 1/2 tsp salt
- 1/8 tsp. ground black pepper

Instructions:
- Place the cooked shredded chicken in a medium sized mixing bowl.
- Place the basil, avocado, olive oil, low sodium salt and ground black pepper in a food processor and blend until smooth.
- Pour the avocado and basil mixture into the mixing bowl with the shredded chicken and toss well to coat.
- Taste and add additional low sodium salt and ground black pepper if desired. Keep in the fridge until ready to serve.

CHINESE DIVINE SALAD

Ingredients:

Salad:
- 1 small head (or 4 cups) savoy cabbage, finely shredded -
- 1 cup carrot, julienned (about 1 large carrot)

- 1/4 cup scallions, trimmed and julienned (about 3 scallions)
- 1/4 cup radishes, julienned
- 1/4 cup fresh cilantro, chopped
- 1/4 cup fresh mint, chopped
- cups cooked chicken or turkey

Vinaigrette:
- 2 tablespoons coconut or rice vinegar
- salt to taste
- 2 tablespoons sesame oil
- 1 chipotle pepper
- 1/2 teaspoon chili flakes
- 1 clove garlic, crushed
- 1 teaspoon fresh ginger, grated
- Stevia to taste

Instructions:

- Combine cabbage, carrots, scallions and radishes. Top with chicken, cilantro and mint and set aside.

- Combine the vinaigrette ingredients. Taste to see if it needs any adjustments. If it is too spicy, you can add more lime juice to counteract it.

- Drizzle salad with vinaigrette & enjoy

DIVINE SALAD SURPRISE

Ingredients:
- 1/2 lb leftover chicken or turkey, cooked and chopped
- 2 cups Shredded lettuce
- 3 tbsp sliced olives
- 1/2 cup sliced tomatoes
- 1/2 cup sliced red onion
- 1/2 cup sliced Avocado
- 1/2 cup sliced bell peppers
- 2 tbsp divine dressing

Instructions:

Divine Dressing:

- Mix together, 4 Tbsp. chili powder, 1 tsp each garlic powder, onion powder, and oregano, 2 tsp each paprika and cumin, 4 tsp low sodium salt, and 1/8 1/4 tsp red pepper flakes. Add 1 cup olive oil and half cup rice vinegar.
- Assemble all the salad ingredients. Add Divine Dressing, toss well and serve.

AVOCADO SALAD WITH CILANTRO AND LIME

Ingredients:
- 1 cooked Turkey Breast chopped
- 2 avocados, diced
- 2/3 green cabbage, chopped
- 5 green onions (scallions), white and pale green parts, minced
- Juice of 2 limes

- 2 handfuls of fresh cilantro, chopped
- salt to taste
- 1 large English Cucumber

Instructions:

- Mix all ingredients except cucumber -slice it thinly and use it as a base for the salad.

MEXICAN MEDLEY SALAD

Ingredients:

For the Chicken or turkey:

- 1 lb boneless chicken/turkey breasts
- 1 tbsp olive oil
- salt and pepper, to taste

For the Salsa:

- 1 large tomato, quartered
- 1/2 red onion, cut into large chunks
- 1 jalapeno pepper, stem and seeds removed and halved
- 1 garlic clove, peeled
- 1 small bunch of cilantro leaves
- Juice of 1 lime
- salt and pepper, to taste

Instructions:

- Preheat the oven to 375 F. Brush chicken breasts on both sides with olive oil and sprinkle with low sodium salt and pepper. Bake on a baking sheet for 35 to 40 minutes, until no longer pink in the center.

- Add all salsa ingredients to a food processor and pulse using the chopping blade until finely chopped.

- Transfer the salsa to a large bowl and clean out the food processor. You will be using it to shred the chicken.

- Remove chicken from the oven and let it cool. Once cool enough to handle, cut each breast into three or four smaller pieces and add to the food processor. Pulse using the chopping blade until shredded.

- Add chicken to a bowl with salsa and mix well with a fork. Refrigerate for at least two hours until chicken salad is chilled.

ARTICHOKE HEART & TURKEY SALAD RADICCHIO CUPS

Ingredients:

- 1 1/2 cups diced cooked turkey
- 1 cup finely diced red onion
- 1 small carrot julienned and cut into small pieces
- 4-5 artichoke hearts diced

- salt and pepper to taste.
- 6 Radicchio leaves

Instructions:

- Place all ingredients, except the radicchio leaves in a large bowl and combine.

- Place a scoop of salad into each Radicchio cup and serve.

TEMPTING TUNA STUFFED TOMATO

Ingredients:

- 2 large tomatoes
- Lettuce leaves (optional)
- 2 (5 or 6 oz.) cans wild albacore tuna
- 1 stalk celery, chopped
- 1/2 small onion, chopped
- 1/4 tsp. low sodium salt
- 1/4 tsp. ground black pepper

Instructions:

- Wash and dry the tomatoes and remove any stem. Arrange the tomatoes on a plate on top of lettuce leaves (optional).

- Combine the remaining ingredients in a mixing bowl and add additional low sodium salt and/or pepper if desired. Spoon into the tomatoes and serve.

AVOCADO TUNA SALAD

Ingredients:
- 1 avocado
- 2 tbsp lemon juice
- 1 tbsp chopped onion
- 5 ounces cooked or canned wild tuna
- salt and pepper to taste

Instructions:

- Cut the avocado in half and scoop the middle of both avocado halves into a bowl, leaving a shell of avocado flesh about 1/4-inch thick on each half.

- Add lemon juice and onion to the avocado in the bowl and mash together. Add tuna, low sodium salt and pepper, and stir to combine. Taste and adjust if needed. Fill avocado shells with tuna salad and serve.

ITALIAN TUNA BONANZA SALAD

Ingredients:
- 10 sun-dried tomatoes
- (5 oz) can of tuna
- 1-2 ribs of celery, diced finely
- 2 Tablespoons of extra virgin olive oil
- 1 clove garlic, minced
- 2 Tablespoons finely chopped parsley
- 1/2 Tablespoon lemon juice
- salt and pepper to tasteInstructions:

- Prepare the sun-dried tomatoes by softening them in warm water for 30 minutes until soft. Then, pat the tomatoes dry and chop finely.

- Flake the tuna. and mix the tuna together with the chopped tomatoes, celery, extra virgin olive oil, garlic, parsley, and lemon juice. Add low sodium salt and pepper to taste.

ASIAN ASPIRATION SALAD

Ingredients:

- 1 red bell pepper, sliced
- 1 large carrot, cut into matchsticks
- cucumber, halved lengthwise and sliced
- Optional: fresh ginger juice and rice vinegar; boiled eggs

Instructions:

- Mix ingredients and Serve.

TASTY CARROT SALAD

Ingredients:

- 5 carrots, medium
- 1 tsp whole black mustard seeds
- 1/4 tsp. low sodium salt
- 1 tsp. lemon juice
- 2 tbsp . olive oil
- 1 Grated egg

Instructions:

- Trim and peel and grate carrots. In a bowl, toss with salt and set aside.

- In a small heavy pan over medium heat, heat oil. When very hot, add mustard seeds. As soon as the seeds begin to pop, in a few seconds, pour oil and seeds over carrots.

- Add lemon juice and toss. Serve at room temperature or cold. Add Grated egg.

CREAMY CARROT SALAD

Ingredients:
- 1 lb carrots, shredded
- 20 oz crushed pineapple, drained
- 8 oz Coconut milk
- 3/4 cup flaked coconut
- Stevia to taste
- 1 breast of turkey, shredded

Instructions:
- Combine all ingredients, tossing well. Cover and chill.

SEA SCALLOPS SENSATION

Ingredients:

For the dressing:
- 1 tbsp red wine vinegar
- 1 tbsp cider vinegar
- 1 tbsp olive oil
- 1 tsp minced shallots
- 2 drops tbsp stevia

For the salad:
- 2 cups diced cooked and peeled beets
- 12 large sea scallops
- olive oil cooking spray
- salt and pepper to taste
- 1 oz baby arugula
- 8 grape tomatoes, halved

Instructions:

- Cover the beets with water in a medium pot and bring to a boil. Cover and cook over medium-low heat until tender when pierced with a fork, about 50 to 60 minutes. Peel and dice into small cubes; set aside to cool.

- Season scallops with low sodium salt and pepper. Heat a large nonstick pan on a medium-high heat. When the pan is hot, spray with oil and place scallops in the pan. Sear without touching them until the bottom forms a nice caramel colored crust, about 2 to 3 minutes.

- Turn and cook until their centers are still slightly

translucent (you can check this by viewing them from the side), about 1 to 2 more minutes, careful not to overcook. Remove from the pan.

- Make vinaigrette by whisking the dressing ingredients in a small bowl. Toss with the arugula. Evenly divide the arugula between four large plates.

- Top each with 1/2 cup beet, tomato and 3 scallops each. Serve immediately.

PURE DELISH SPINACH SALAD

Ingredients:
- 2 bunches fresh spinach
- 1 bunch scallions, chopped
- juice of 1 lemon
- 1/4 tbsp olive oil
- pepper to taste
- optional: rice vinegar to taste

Instructions:
- Wash spinach well. Drain and chop. After a few minutes, squeeze excess water.

- Add scallions, lemon juice, oil and pepper.

SALSA SALAD

Ingredients:
- 1 bunch of cilantro
- 5-6 roma tomatoes

- 1 small yellow or red onion
- 1 small chili pepper
- 2 ripe avocados.
- A handful of arugula leaves

Instructions:

- Chop cilantro, dice tomatoes, dice onion, finely dice chili pepper, dice avocado.
- After dicing each ingredient add to a large bowl. Add arugula to the bowl and toss.

EASTERN AVOCADO SALAD

Ingredients:

- 2 to 3 lbs. of tomatoes
- 4 avocados
- 4 stalks celery
- 4 bell peppers
- 2 lbs. bok choy stalks and greens

Instructions:

- Dice the tomatoes, celery and the bell peppers. Quarter, peel and dice the avocados.
- Cut up the bok choy. Place all ingredients in a bowl and mix together.

CURRY COCONUT SALAD

Ingredients:

- 2 large ripe tomatoes, peeled, seeded and chopped

- 1 small white onion, grated
- 1/4 tsp. coarsely ground pepper
- 1/2 cup coconut cream
- 1 Tbsp minced fresh parsley
- 1 tsp. curry powder

Instructions:

- Combine tomatoes, onion and pepper; cover and chill for 3 hours. Combine coconut cream, parsley and curry; cover and chill for 3 hours.
- To serve, spoon tomato mixture into small bowls and top each with a spoonful of coconut cream mixture.

JALAPENO SALSA

Ingredients:

- 1 jalapeno pepper seeded and chopped fine
- 2 large ripe tomatoes, peeled and chopped
- 1 medium onion, minced
- 1 tbsp olive oil
- juice of 1 lemon
- 1/2 tsp dried oregano
- pepper to taste

Instructions:

- Combine all ingredients and mix well. Refrigerate covered until ready to eat.

BEET SPROUT DIVINE SALAD

Ingredients:

- 1/2 pound Brussels sprouts, trimmed, and cut in half lengthwise
- 4 small red beets, tops trimmed to 1/2-inch, washed and cut in half lengthwise
- 4 tablespoons + 1/3 cup extra virgin olive oil
- 1 tablespoon paleo Dijon mustard
- Stevia to taste
- 1 Squeeze of lemon juice
- Salt & pepper to taste
- 1 small red onion thinly sliced into ringsInstructions:
- Preheat the oven to 350.Pour 2 tablespoons of olive oil in a baking dish. Toss the Brussels sprouts in the oil; sprinkle them with low sodium salt and pepper and roast them for 20 minutes.

- Turn them once during cooking. They are done when a small knife easily pierces them.

- Pour 2 tablespoons of the olive oil on a sheet of aluminum foil and place it on a baking sheet.

- Toss the beet halves in the olive oil. Sprinkle them with low sodium salt and pepper and, keeping them in a single layer, fold and seal the foil over them. Bake on the baking sheet until a knife easily pierces them.

- When cool enough to handle, peel the beets and cut them into 1/4-inch slices.

- Meanwhile combine the 1/3 cup olive oil,

mustard, stevia, lemon juice and low sodium salt and pepper in a small bowl.

- Toss the Ingredients, add the dressing and serve at room temperature.

DIVINE CARROT SALAD

Ingredients:
- 2 tablespoons fresh lemon juice
- 1 tablespoon Olive oil
- 1 pressed garlic clove
- 1-1/2 pound carrots, peeled and rectangle and lightly steamed

Instructions:
- Mix dressing ingredients in a small bowl. Add carrots; toss to mix.
- Let stand at room temperature for one hour and then serve.

CAULIFLOWER COUSCOUS

Ingredients:
- 1/2 Lbs cauliflower florets
- 1/2 cup parsley (finely chopped)
- 1/2 cup fresh mint (Finely chopped)
- 1/2 cup chopped red onion
- 1 cucumber finely cubed
- 5 Tbsp fresh lime juice
- 1 Tbsp olive oil

- 1 tsp low sodium salt
- 1 tsp black pepper

Instructions:

- In a food processor pulse cauliflower until it looks like rice. Set aside.
- In a food processor- blend parsley, mint, onion, lime juice, olive oil, salt and pepper into a smooth paste. Pour over cauliflower and cucumber and blend well.

MUSHROOM SALAD

Ingredients:

- 2/3 cup olive oil
- 1/3 cup fresh lemon juice
- One tablespoon red wine vinegar
- 1 tsp dried thyme
- pepper and garlic powder to taste
- 1 pound fresh mushrooms, thinly sliced
- 1/4 cup minced parsley
- Rucola leaves

Instructions:

- Combine all ingredients except the mushrooms, parsley and greens, and mix well.

- Add the mushrooms and toss with 2 forks. Cover and let stand at room temperature.

- At serving time, drain and sprinkle with the parsley. Pile in a serving dish lined with greens.

SKINNY SWEET POTATO SALAD

Ingredients:
- 2 small sweet potatoes
- 1 tablespoon olive oil extra virgin
- 1 teaspoon mustard powder
- 4 celery stalks, sliced 1/4-inch thick
- 1 small red bell pepper, cut into 1/4-inch dice
- 2 scallions, finely chopped
- salt and pepper
- 1/2 cup coarsely chopped toasted pecans
- Chopped fresh chives

Instructions:
- Preheat the oven to 400°F. Wrap each sweet potato in foil and bake for 1 hour.

- Unwrap; let cool. Peel; cut into 3/4-inch chunks.

- In a large bowl, mix oil and mustard. Add sweet potatoes, celery, red pepper and scallions; toss gently.

- Season to taste with low sodium salt and pepper. Cover and refrigerate for about 1 hour. Fold in pecans and sprinkle with chives.

BROWNIE TREATS

Ingredients:
- 1 1/2 cups walnuts

- A pinch of salt
- 1 tsp vanilla
- 1/3 cup unsweetened cocoa powder

Instructions:

- Add walnuts and low sodium salt to a blender or food processor. Mix until the walnuts are finely ground.

- Add the vanilla, and cocoa powder to the blender. Mix well until everything is combined.

- With the blender still running, add a couple drops of water at a time to make the mixture stick together.

- Using a spatula, transfer the mixture into a bowl. Using your hands, form small round balls, rolling in your palm.

ROSE BANANA DELICIOUS BROWNIES

Ingredients:

- 2 red beets, cooked
- 2 bananas
- 2 eggs
- 1/2 cup unsweetened cocoa powder
- 1/3 cup almond flour
- 1 tsp baking powder
- 2 tablespoons crushes mixed nuts
- Stevia to taste

Instructions:

- Combine all ingredients in a food processor, and blend until smooth.

- Stir in the nut bits. Pour into a well-greased pan. Bake at 325 F for about 40 minutes.

PRISTINE PUMPKIN DIVINE

Ingredients:
- 2 cups blanched almond flour
- 1 cup flaxseed meal
- 2 teaspoons ground cinnamon (optional)
- Stevia to taste
- teaspoon low sodium salt
- 1 egg
- 1 cup pumpkin puree
- 1 tablespoon vanilla extract

Instructions:

- Mix together the almond flour, flaxseed meal, cinnamon, and low sodium salt.

- In a separate bowl, whisk the egg, pumpkin and vanilla extract using a rubber spatula. Gently mix dry and wet ingredients to form a batter, being careful not to over mix or the batter will get oily and dense.

- Spoon the batter onto a 9-inch pan lined with parchment paper or grease the pan ; bake at 350°F until a toothpick inserted into the center comes out clean, approximately 25 minutes.

SECRET BROWNIES

Ingredients:
- 1 c. raw almonds
- 1/2 c. raw cashews
- 4-5 Tbs. cocoa powder
- 1 Tbs. cashew butter
- Stevia to taste

Instructions:

- Combine all ingredients in the food processor. Process until somewhat smooth.
- Press into a glass baking dish. Chill until ready to serve.

SPINACH BROWNIES

Ingredients:

- 1 1/2 cups frozen chopped spinach
- 6 oz sugar free chocolate
- 1 cup extra virgin coconut oil
- 1 cup coconut oil
- 6 eggs
- Stevia to taste
- 1 cup cocoa powder
- 1 Tsp vanilla pod
- 1 tsp baking soda
- 1 tsp low sodium salt
- 1 tsp cream of tartar
- pinch cinnamon

Instructions:

- Preheat the oven to 325 F. Line a baking pan with wax paper or use a silicone baking pan.

- Melt coconut oil and chocolate together over low heat on the stove top or medium power in the microwave. Add vanilla and stir to incorporate. Let cool.

- Mix cocoa powder, baking soda, cream of tartar, low sodium salt and cinnamon. Blend spinach, egg, together in a food processor or blender, until completely smooth.

- Add coconut oil to the food processor and process until fully incorporated. Add melted chocolate mixture and 3 or 4 drops of stevia liquid to egg mixture slowly and process/blending constantly.

- Mix in dry ingredients and process/stir to fully incorporate. Pour batter into the prepared baking pan and spread out with a spatula.
- Bake for 40 minutes. Cool completely in the pan. Cut into squares. Enjoy!

CHOCO-COCONUT BROWNIES

Ingredients:

- 6 Tablespoons of coconut oil
- 6 oz of Sugar free Chocolate
- 2 Tablespoons of Coconut Flour
- 1 cup of Unsweetened Cocoa Powder
- 2 Eggs
- 1 teaspoon of Baking Soda
- 1 teaspoon of low sodium salt
- Extra coconut oil for pan greasing
- Stevia to taste

Instructions:

- Preheat the oven to 350 F. Grease an 8x8 baking pan and line with parchment paper.

- Gently melt the semisweet chocolate and oil. Stir in unsweetened cocoa powder.
- Sift together the superfine coconut flour, baking soda, stevia and low sodium salt. Beat the eggs and add the dry ingredients. Beat until combined
- Add the rest of the wet ingredients and beat until incorporated. Pour the batter into the lined pan.
- Bake for 25-30 minutes at 350 F until a toothpick inserted into the center of the batter comes out clean.

COCO - WALNUT BROWNIE BITES

Ingredients:
- 2/3 cup raw walnut halves and pieces
- 1/3 cup unsweetened cocoa powder
- 1 tablespoon vanilla extract
- 1 to 2 tablespoons coconut milk
- 2/3 cups shredded unsweetened coconut

Instructions:
- Pulse coconut in a food processor for 30 seconds to a minute to form coconut crumbs. Remove from the food processor and set aside.

- Add unsweetened cocoa powder and walnuts to the food processor, blend until walnuts become fine crumb.

- Place in the food processor the cocoa walnut crumbs. Add vanilla. Process until mixture starts to combine.

- Add coconut milk. You will know the consistency is right when the dough combines into a ball in the middle of the food processor.

- Transfer dough to a bowl and cover with plastic wrap. Refrigerate for at least 2 hours. Cold dough is much easier to work with.

- Roll the dough balls in coconut crumbs, pressing the crumbs gently into the ball.

BEST EVER BLUEBERRY SURPRISE CAKE

Ingredients:

Bottom Fruit Layer
- 2 tbsp coconut oil, melted
- 1 cup blueberries
- 2 tbsp walnut pieces
- Stevia to taste
- 1 tsp ground cinnamon.

Top Cake Layer
- 2 eggs, beaten.
- Stevia to taste
- 1 cup unsweetened coconut milk, or unsweetened almond milk.
- 1 tsp organic vanilla extract
- 1 tsp baking soda.
- 1 tsp apple cider vinegar.
- 1 cup blueberries
- 1 cup coconut flour

Instructions:

- Preheat the oven to 350 F, and lightly grease a 9 inch cake pan.

- Place 2 tbsp coconut oil into a cake pan, and put the pan into the preheating oven for a couple minutes to melt butter or oil. Once melted, make sure butter or oil is evenly distributed all over the bottom of the pan.

- Sprinkle 2-4 drops of stevia sweetener all over the melted oil.Sprinkle 1 tsp cinnamon on top of the sweetener layer.

- Layer banana slices or blueberries on top of butter. Add optional walnut pieces to the fruit layer. Set aside.

- In a large mixing bowl combine all the "top cake layer" ingredients except for the coconut flour. Mix thoroughly, then add the coconut flour and mix well, scraping sides of bowl, and breaking up any coconut flour clumps.

- Spoon cake batter on top of the fruit layer in the cake pan . Spread cake batter evenly across the entire pan. Bake for 25 minutes or until the top of the cake is browned and the center is set.

- Remove from the oven and let cool completely. Use a butter knife between the cake and the edge of the pan and slide around to loosen the cake from the pan. Turn the cake pan upside down onto a large plate or serving platter.

CHOCO COOKIE DELIGHT

Ingredients:
- 1/2 cup dark chocolate sugar free chips
- 1/2 cup coconut milk (thick fat from top of can)
- 2 eggs
- 1 cup almond flour
- pinch of low sodium salt
- 1/2 teaspoon vanilla extract
- 1/4 teaspoon baking powder

Vanilla glaze:
- 1/2 cup coconut butter, liquid
- Stevia to taste
- 1/2 teaspoon vanilla extract

Chocolate Glaze:
- 1/2 cup chocolate chips
- Stevia powder for decoration

Instructions:
- Place a small saucepan over low heat and melt your chocolate and coconut milk together.

- While melting, place your 2 eggs in a stand mixer with the whisk, or use a hand mixer with the whisk and beat your eggs until they are fluffy, about 1 minute

- Add your coconut milk and chocolate to your eggs and mix well. Stir in your almond flour, low sodium salt, vanilla extract and baking powder.

- Mix well ensuring everything is combined .Pipe your batter into the cookie wells ensuring you fill higher than the halfway point.

- Remove from the cookie maker, gently insert the sticks and place everything in the freezer for 30-45 minutes.

- Combine your coconut butter, stevia, and vanilla extract in a small glass to make it easy to dip.

- You can keep this glass in hot water to keep the glaze more liquidy to make the dipping easier.

- Melt your chocolate chips over a double boiler and keep the heat low and then liquid - then spread over cooled cookies!

CHOCO TRIPLE DELIGHT

Ingredients:

Cake:

- 1 cup almond flour (or 3 oz ground raw pumpkin seeds for nut-free version)
- tbsp Raw Cacao Powder
- 1 tbsp coconut flour
- 1 tsp baking powder
- 1/2 tsp baking soda
- 1/8th tsp Stevia
- 1 tbsp melted coconut oil
- Pinch of low sodium salt
- 1 large pastured egg
- 1 tbsp coconut milk
- 1 tsp pure vanilla extract
- 1 oz 80% cocoa bar, chopped

Chocolate Drizzle:

- 1 tbsp coconut cream concentrate, warmed
- 1 tbsp water (or coconut milk)
- 1 tbsp Cacao powder
- 1/2 tbsp pure vanilla extract
- Stevia to taste

Instructions:

- Preheat the oven to 350 degrees F. Oil the sides of the cake pan.

- Line the bottom of the pan with parchment

paper and set aside. In a medium bowl, add dry ingredients.

- Add remaining ingredients (except nuts and optional salt) to dry ingredients and mix.
- Press into a cake pan. Sprinkle with nuts. Bake for 11-14 minutes. DO NOT OVER BAKE! Remove from the oven and serve warm or allow to cool.
- Top with Chocolate Drizzle.

Chocolate Drizzle:

- In a small bowl, blend coconut cream concentrate and water until smooth.
- Add cacao powder, vanilla and stevia. Whisk until creamy.

PEACH AND ALMOND CAKE

Ingredients:

- 2 whole peaches
- 3 cups almond meal
- 6 eggs
- Stevia to taste
- 1 tsp baking soda

Instructions:

- Cover the peaches in water in a saucepan and boil for about 2 hours. Preheat the oven to 350 F and line the bottom of a pan with baking paper.
- Lightly beat the eggs. Blend the eggs and peaches thoroughly in a food processor.

Add the rest of the ingredients to the food processor, blending thoroughly. Pour mixture into the lined tin and bake for roughly an hour.

APPLE CINNAMON WALNUT BONANZA

Ingredients:

For the cake:
- 1 cup almond flour
- 2 tablespoons coconut flour
- Stevia to taste
- 1 tablespoon cinnamon
- 1 teaspoon baking soda
- 1/4 teaspoon low sodium salt
- 1 tablespoon coconut butter, plus more for greasing the pan
- 3 eggs
- 1/2 cup cream from a can of refrigerated coconut milk
- 1 teaspoon vanilla
- 1 cup grated apple (about 1 large apple)

For the topping:
- 1 1/2 cups walnuts (or pecans, if you prefer)
- 1/2 cup almond flour
- 2 tablespoons melted coconut butter
- Stevia to taste
- 1 tablespoon cinnamon
- pinch low sodium salt

Instructions:

- Preheat your oven to 350°F and grease a baking dish. Pulse the walnuts in a food processor 10-12 times or until they are coarse crumbs.
- Add the remaining ingredients and pulse 2-3 more times until combined. Set aside.
- Wipe out and dry the bowl of your food processor and add your dry cake ingredients Pulse a few times to mix.
- Cut the tablespoon of butter into smaller chunks and add it to the dry ingredients. Pulse until it's similar to if you were making a pie crust.
- In a small bowl, mix your wet cake ingredients and whisk until well combined. Stir in grated apple.
- Add to the food processor and mix until combined. Scrape down the sides once or twice to make sure it's well mixed.
- Pour into the prepared baking dish and sprinkle the topping over, as evenly as you can.
- Bake for 30-35 minutes, or until a toothpick inserted into the center comes out clean

CHESTNUT-CACAO CAKE

Ingredients:
- 1 cup + 1 heaping tablespoon chestnut flour
- 1/2 cup almond flour
- 2 eggs, separate
- 1/2 teaspoon cream of tartar
- 1/2 cup raw cacao powder
- Stevia to taste
- 3/4 cup coconut milk
- 1/2 teaspoon baking soda
- Crushed chestnuts

Instructions:
- Preheat the oven to 350 F. Grease a pie/tart pan.

- In a clean mixing bowl, beat the egg whites and cream of tartar until stiff peaks form. Set aside. In another mixing bowl, cream the egg yolks, chestnut flour, ground almonds, stevia, raw cacao, baking soda and coconut milk.

- Fold in the egg whites and blend until the white is no longer showing. Pour into the pie/tart mold.

- Sprinkle with crushed chestnuts, if desired. Bake for 35-40 minutes on the middle rack.

EXTRA DARK CHOCO DELIGHT

Ingredients:
- 1 egg
- 1 ripe avocado
- 1 cup full fat canned coconut milk
- 1 tbsp cacao powder
- 1 tbsp carob powder
- pinch low sodium salt
- pinch cinnamon
- 1 scoop vanilla flavored hemp protein powder
- 1 tbsp raw hazelnuts
- 3 tbsp unsweetened shredded coconut

Instructions:
- Add the egg, avocado and coconut milk to a small food processor and process smooth and creamy.

- Add cacao powder, carob powder, low sodium salt, cinnamon and protein powder and process again until well combined and creamy.

- Add hazelnuts and shredded coconut and give a few extra spins until the hazelnuts are reduced to tiny little pieces.

- Serve immediately or refrigerate until ready to serve.

- Garnish with a little dollop of coconut cream and cacao nibs or shredded coconut and crushed hazelnuts.

NUT BUTTER TRUFFLES

Ingredients:
- 3 tablespoons sunflower seed butter
- 1 tablespoon coconut oil
- 2 teaspoons vanilla extract
- 1 cup almond flour
- 1 tablespoon flaxseed meal
- pinch of low sodium salt
- 1 cup sugar free dark chocolate chips
- 1 tablespoon cacao butter
- chopped almonds (optional)

Instructions:
- Add sunflower seed butter, coconut oil, vanilla, almond flour, flaxseed meal and low sodium salt to a large bowl.

- Using your hands, mix until all ingredients are incorporated. Roll the dough into 1-inch balls and place them on a sheet of parchment paper and refrigerate for 30 minutes.

- Melt the chocolate chips in a double boiler along with the cacao butter. Dip each truffle in the melted chocolate, one at the time, and place them back on the pan with parchment paper.

- Top with chopped almonds and refrigerate until the chocolate is firm.

FETCHING FUDGE

Ingredients:
- 1 cup coconut butter
- 1/4 cup coconut oil
- 1/4 cup cocoa
- 1/4 cup cocoa powder + 1 Tbsp
- Stevia to taste
- 1 tsp vanilla

Instructions:
- In the pot, gently melt the cocoa butter on low ; when it is half melted add the butter, the coconut oil and the coconut spread and gently mix with the whisk as it melts.

- Add vanilla, and stevia and whisk in well . Add the cocoa powder and whisk in well

- Be sure to take the pot off the heat when the fat is melted and keep whisking until it is smooth and all the lumps are out .

- Pour into the pan that is lined with parchment paper . Refrigerate for 1 - 2 hours; When solid, pull the parchment paper out of the pan, put the block of fudge on a flat surface and cut into small squares

CHOCO - ALMOND DELIGHTS

Ingredients:
- 1 c. toasted hazelnuts
- 1 c. raw almonds
- 2/3 c. raw almond butter

- 5 Tbs. raw cacao powder (or unsweetened cocoa powder)
- 1/2 tsp. vanilla extract
- 1/4 c. unsweetened, shredded coconut

Instructions:

- Combine all the ingredients, except for the coconut, in the food processor. Whir until smooth.
- Line a muffin tin with plastic wrap. Spoon dollops of the sweet mixture into the lined tin cups and form into "mounds."

- Freeze until well formed. Remove mounds from plastic and tin and flip for presentation. Sprinkle with shredded coconut.

CHOCO CUPS

Ingredients:

- 2 eggs
- Stevia to taste
- 1/3 cup coconut flour
- 1/4 cup cacao powder
- 1/2 teaspoon baking soda
- 1/4 cup coconut oil (melted in microwave)
- 1/4 cup cacao butter (melted in microwave)

For topping:

- 1 can coconut cream (chilled in fridge overnight)
- Cacao nibs to decorate.

Instructions:

- Heat oven to 338F. Grease 10 muffin pans with

coconut oil.

- Beat eggs with electric beaters. Add coconut flour, baking soda and cacao powder.Beat well and add stevia . Add melted coconut oil, cacao butter and mix.
- Spoon mixture into 10 greased muffin pans. Bake for 12-15 minutes until risen and top springs back. Beat the solid coconut cream with electric beaters until creamy. Add honey to taste if you wish. Pipe coconut cream onto top of cakes.

CHOCO COCO COOKIES

Ingredients:

- Stevia powder - to taste
- 1 cup coconut flour
- 1 cup coconut oil
- 1 cup coconut milk, (from the can)
- 2 Teaspoons vanilla extract
- 1/2 Teaspoon low sodium salt
- 2 cups finely shredded coconut
- 1 cup large flake coconut
- 1 cup dark sugar free chocolate chips

Instructions:

- In a large saucepan, combine the coconut oil, and coconut milk. Bring the mixture to a boil, and boil for 2-3 minutes.

- Remove from the heat and add the vanilla, low sodium salt, and coconut flour and coconut. Stir to combine. Add the chocolate chips and combine, stirring as little as possible to keep the chunks intact.

- Portion the cookie on a parchment lined baking sheet and let it set up.

APPLE SPICE SPECTACULAR

Ingredients:

- 1 cup unsweetened almond butter
- Stevia to taste
- 1 egg
- 1 tsp baking soda
- 1/2 tsp salt
- 1/2 apple, diced
- 1 tsp cinnamon
- 1/4 tsp ground cloves
- 1/8 tsp nutmeg
- 1 tsp grated fresh ginger

Instructions:

- Preheat the oven to 350 degrees F. In a large bowl, combine almond butter, stevia, egg, baking soda, and low sodium salt until well incorporated. Add apple, spices, and ginger and stir to combine.

- Spoon batter onto a baking sheet about 1-2 inches apart from each other, they'll spread a bit.

- Bake for about 10 minutes. Remove cookies and let cool on pan for about 5-10 minutes. Then finish cooling on a cooling rack.

ABSOLUTE ALMOND BITES

Ingredients:

- 1/2 cups almond flour
- 1/4 teaspoon low sodium salt
- 1/4 teaspoon baking soda (gluten-free, if necessary)
- 1/8 teaspoon cinnamon
- 2 tablespoons melted coconut oil
- Stevia to taste
- 1 1/4 teaspoon vanilla extract
- 1/4 teaspoon almond extract or almond flavoring
- 12 to 15 whole almonds; sprouted or soaked and dehydrated

Instructions:

- Preheat the oven to 325°F. Line a baking sheet with parchment paper.

- In a medium bowl combine almond flour, low sodium salt, baking soda, and cinnamon. Mix well, breaking up any lumps.

- In a small bowl, place coconut oil, vanilla, almond extract or flavoring. Whisk until well combined.

- Add wet ingredients to dry ingredients and stir until combined...add stevia Roll level-tablespoon-sized (using a measuring spoon) portions of dough into balls and place on a baking sheet.Flatten slightly with the heel of your hand and press one almond into the center of each cookie.

- Bake for 15 to 17 minutes or until light golden brown. Allow to cool on a baking sheet for a few minutes before transferring to the cooling rack.

EASTERN SPICE DELIGHTS

Ingredients:
- 1 3/4 cups + 4 tbsp almond meal
- 1/8 tsp low sodium salt
- 3/4 tsp ground ginger
- 3/4 tsp cinnamon
- 1/4 tsp ground cloves
- 1/4 tsp cardamom
- 1/8 tsp nutmeg
- 1/2 cup coconut oil (in solid form)
- Stevia to taste
- 1 tsp vanilla extract

Instructions:
- Preheat the oven to 350 F.

- Combine all the dry ingredients in a large bowl. In a small bowl, mix together the oil, maple syrup, and vanilla until completely blended.

- Pour the wet ingredients over the dry ingredients and mix well. Drop the cookie dough on a cookie sheet. Bake for 10-12 minutes.

BERRY ICE CREAM AND ALMOND DELIGHT

Ingredients:

For the Ice Cream:
- 1 can full fat coconut milk
- Stevia to taste
- 1 tbsp vanilla
- 1 cup fresh strawberries cut into fourths

For the crisp:
- 1/3 cup almond flour
- 1 tbsp sunflower seed butter (or almond butter)
- 1/2 tsp vanilla
- 1 tbsp honey
- salt to taste

Instructions:

- Combine coconut milk and vanilla together in a small saucepan over medium heat and stir until ingredients are well combined.

- Transfer milk mixture to a small bowl and place in the freezer for two hours.Next, add strawberries to a small saucepan and bring to a low boil.

- Turn heat to medium-low and allow to cook until they start breaking down into a sauce-like mixture, leaving small chunks.

- Place strawberries in the refrigerator while the ice cream hardens. Combine all ingredients and mix until you get a "crumble' consistency.

- Place crisp in the refrigerator until ready to use. After two hours, place milk mixture into your ice cream maker along with the strawberries and use as directed.

- When ice cream is ready, scoop and serve with crisp sprinkled on top.

CREAMY CARAMEL ICE CREAM

Ingredients:

Instant Caramel Topping:
- 2 heaped tablespoons of hulled tahini
- Stevia to taste
- 2 tablespoons of coconut milk
- 1/2 teaspoon of vanilla

Instant Ice Cream:
- 2 frozen bananas, chopped
- 4 tablespoons coconut milk
- 1 teaspoon of vanilla

Instructions:

- Spoon the tahini and stevia into a cup and stir with a fork to combine. Mix in the coconut milk and vanilla.

- Place the ingredients into a food processor or blender, blend until the mixture is an ice cream consistency.

- Spoon the ice cream into bowls, drizzle generously with the caramel topping, sprinkle with low sodium salt if you desire. Enjoy!

CHEEKY CHERRY ICE

Ingredients:
- 14oz. can Coconut Milk
- Stevia to taste
- 1 tsp. vanilla extract
- 2 cups fresh cherries, pitted and diced

Instructions:
- In a large bowl, combine coconut milk, stevia and vanilla and stir well. Chill for 1-2 hours.
- Transfer to ice-cream maker and process according to manufacturer

directions. Add diced cherries to the mixture during the last 5-10 minutes of processing.

CHOCO - COCONUT BERRY ICE

Ingredients:
- Coconut ice cream
- 4 oz sugar free dark chocolate - 75% cacao content
- 1 cup coconut milk
- 2 cups fresh berries

Instructions:
- Combine the chocolate and coconut milk in a sauce pan and melt, stirring over low heat.

- When the chocolate mixture is completely smooth, pour the chocolate over the ice cream and stir to create 'ripples'. If your ice cream is thoroughly frozen, soften in the fridge for 20 minutes before stirring in the chocolate.

- Serve immediately with the fresh berries, or freeze for an additional 3-4 hours for a firmer texture.

CREAMY BERRY PIE

Ingredients:

Crust:
- 2 cups almonds
- 1 Teaspoon cinnamon
- 1 cup honey
- 2 Tablespoons coconut oil
- 1 tablespoon lemon zest
- 1 Teaspoon almond extract
- A pinch of low sodium salt

Filling:
- Teaspoons plant-based gelatin, dissolved in 2 Tablespoons hot water
- 1 cup freshly squeezed lemon juice
- Stevia to taste
- 1 can coconut milk, chilled
- 2 cups blueberries for serving

Instructions:

- Place the almonds and cinnamon in a food processor and pulse until your desired texture is reached. Add the rest of the crust ingredients and pulse until a sticky dough forms. Pat the crust into a pie plate, (use water to keep your hands from sticking to the crust)

- Mix the gelatin and water together. Stir to dissolve and immediately add the lemon juice. If the gelatin gets clumpy, place the mixture over hot water until it melts again.

- Pour the coconut milk into an electric mixer, add the stevia and whip on high until peaks form, about 15 minutes. Add the gelatin mixture to the whipped cream. Pour the filling into the crust. Chill for at least 4 hours until set, and serve with lots of berries!

PEACHY CREAMY PEACHES

Ingredients:
- 2 medium ripe peaches cut in half with pit removed
- 1 tsp vanilla
- 1 can coconut milk, refrigerated
- 1/4 cup chopped walnuts
- Cinnamon (to taste)

Instructions:
- Place peaches on the grill with the cut side down first. Grill on medium-low heat until soft, about 3-5

minutes on each side.

- Scoop cream off the top of the can of chilled coconut milk. Whip together coconut cream and vanilla with a handheld mixer. Drizzle over each peach. Top with cinnamon and chopped walnuts to garnish.

SPICED APPLE BAKE

Ingredients:
- 2 large apples
- 1/4 cup walnuts
- 1/4 tablespoon nutmeg
- 1/4 tablespoon cinnamon
- 1/4 tablespoon ground cloves

Instructions:
- Preheat the oven to 350 degrees F.

- Slice the very top and very bottom off of each apple. Core both apples to the bottom, but not all the way through.

- Mix spices, walnuts, and raisins in a small bowl. Pour half of the spice mixture into each apple.

- Place on a baking sheet and bake for 20-25 minutes, or until the apples are soft. I like to pour any remaining sauce mixture into the bottom of the pan so the apples can soak up the flavors.

SEXY DESSERT PAN

Ingredients:

Crust:
- 1/2 cups pecans
- 3/4 cup dates
- 1 tbsp coconut oil

Second Layer:
- 2/3 cup cashew butter
- 1/3 cup palm shortening
- 1 tsp apple cider vinegar
- 1/2 tsp lemon juice
- Pinch low sodium salt

Third Layer:
- 1 cup coconut flour
- 1 cup coconut milk
- Stevia to taste
- 1 tsp vanilla extract

Fourth Layer:
- 1/2 cup coconut milk
- 1/2 cup coconut butter
- 1/2 cup cacao powder
- tbsp honey

Fifth Layer:
- 1/2 cup coconut butter
- 1/4 cup coconut milk
- Stevia to taste

Sixth Layer:

- Grated dark sugar free chocolate

Instructions:

- Roughly chop the pecans then pit and chop the dates. Load both into a food processor and pulse until ground but still crumbly. Transfer to a bowl and work in the coconut oil, then press the sticky mixture into a single smooth layer at the bottom of a square cake pan.

- Transfer to the refrigerator to chill while you begin the second layer. To make the second layer, combine its ingredients very well in a medium mixing bowl. Spoon over the chilled crust, smoothing as much as possible with the back of a spoon. Place the pan back in the fridge.

- To make the third layer, mix its ingredients together in a mixing bowl and then spoon over the chilled, hardened second layer. Smooth as much as possible, then chill.

- Add the fourth layer by combining its ingredients and then layering it into the pan in the same way as the previous layers.

- For the fifth layer, mix the coconut shortening, coconut milk and stevia with a hand mixer until very smooth and spoon over the chilled fourth layer. Before placing the pan back into the refrigerator after adding the fifth layer, grate very dark chocolate over the top to the depth of your preference.

- Chill the pan for an additional half hour or more, then slice with a sharp knife and serve.

PRETTY PUMPKIN DELIGHTS

Ingredients:

For Crust:
- 1 cup hazelnuts
- 1 tbsp coconut oil
- pinch of low sodium salt
- Stevia to taste

For Filling:
- 1 cup cooked pumpkin puree
- 1/2 cup coconut
- 1 tbsp coconut oil
- Stevia to taste
- 1/2 tsp vanilla extract
- 1/4 tsp cinnamon powder
- 1/4 tsp ginger powder
- 1/8 tsp allspice
- 1/8 tsp clove powder

For Chocolate Drizzle:
- 1 TBSP coconut butter
- 1 TBSP coconut oil
- 2 TBSP raw cacao
- Stevia to taste

- a pinch or 2 of low sodium salt

Instructions:

- Line muffin tins with paper liners. Process all crust ingredients in a food processor. Spoon 1 and 1/2 tsp of mixture into each of the 24 mini cups. Use your thumb to press down the mixture firmly to create a solid bottom layer. Place in the freezer to harden.

- Melt coconut butter and coconut oil in a double boiler. Remove from heat and add the rest of the filling ingredients. Remove crusts from the freezer and spoon filling over them. Return to the freezer to harden, at least 2 hours.

- Melt coconut butter and coconut oil in a double boiler. Remove from heat and add the rest of the drizzle ingredients. Allow to cool slightly to thicken. Pour into a small plastic bag, cut a small hole in the corner, and drizzle over treats.

MACADAMIA PINEAPPLE BONANZA

Ingredients:

Crust:
- 1 cup almond flour
- 2 tablespoons raw cacao powder
- 1 cup macadamia nuts
- 1 teaspoon vanilla extract
- Stevia to taste
- 1 teaspoons coconut oil, melted

Filling:
- 2 eggs
- cup fresh pineapple, chopped
- 1 cup shredded coconut, unsweetened
- 1 tablespoon fresh lime juice
- 1 tablespoon vanilla extract
- Stevia to taste
- 1 cup almond flour
- A pinch of low sodium salt

Instructions:

- In a large bowl, mix the almond flour and cacao powder. Chop the macadamia nuts in a food processor and add it to the bowl.

- Add vanilla extract and coconut oil to the dry mixture and using your hands, mix to combine ingredients. Spread the mixture evenly on the bottom of an 8x8-inch pan lined with parchment paper.

- In a large bowl beat the 2 eggs. Mix in the pineapple, 1 cup of shredded coconut, lime juice, vanilla and stevia.

- Gently mix in the almond flour and low sodium salt with rubber spatula. Pour mixture over the crust and sprinkle top with remaining shredded coconut. Bake at 350°F for approximately 20 minutes

LEMONY LEMON DELIGHTS

Ingredients:

Crust:
- 1 cup almond flour
- 1/4 cup almond butter
- Stevia to taste
- 1 tbsp coconut butter
- 1 tsp vanilla
- 1/2 tsp baking powder
- 1/4 tsp low sodium salt

Filling:
- 2 eggs
- Stevia to taste
- 1/4 cup lemon juice
- 1/2 tbsp coconut flour
- 1 tbsp lemon zest, finely grated
- Pinch of low sodium salt

Instructions:

- Preheat the oven to 350 F. Coat a baking dish with coconut oil or butter. Combine all crust ingredients in a food processor until a "crumble" forms.

- Press the crust evenly into the bottom of the pan. Using a fork, prick a few holes into the crust.

- Bake for 10 minutes. While the crust is baking, combine all filling ingredients in a food processor until well incorporated.

- Remove crust from oven and pour filling evenly over top. Continue to bake for 15-20 minutes. Cool completely on wire rack.

BANANA NUT BREAD

Ingredients:
- 2 bananas, mashed
- 2 eggs
- 1/2 cup almond butter
- 1/4 cup coconut oil, melted
- 1 tsp vanilla extract
- 1/2 cup almond flour
- 1/2 cup coconut flour
- 1 tsp cinnamon
- 1 tsp baking soda
- 1/4 tsp low sodium salt
- 1/2 cup chopped walnuts

Instructions:
- Preheat the oven to 350 degrees F. Line a loaf pan with parchment paper. In a large bowl, add the mashed bananas, eggs, almond butter, coconut oil, and vanilla. Use a hand blender to combine.

- In a separate bowl, mix together the almond flour, coconut flour, cinnamon, baking soda, and low sodium salt.

- Blend the dry ingredients into the wet mixture, scraping down the sides with a spatula. Fold in the walnuts.

- Pour the batter into the loaf pan in an even layer. Bake for 50-60 minutes, until a toothpick inserted into the center comes out clean. Place the bread on a cooling rack and allow to cool before slicing.

BERRY SMOOTHIE

Ingredients:
- 1 cup frozen blueberries or 1 cup fresh blueberries
- 15 oz coconut milk
- Stevia to taste
- 1 scoop of hemp protein
- 1 teaspoon cinnamon (optional)

Instructions:
- Place all ingredients into a blender. Blend until mixed thoroughly.
- Serve right away.

COCONUT BERRY SMOOTHIE

Ingredients:
- 1 Cup Frozen Blackberries
- 1 Frozen Banana
- 1 teaspoon Chia Seeds
- 1 Inch Piece Of Fresh Ginger
- 1 cup Coconut Milk
- 1 scoop of hemp protein
- 2 Tablespoons Toasted Coconut

Instructions:
- Combine all the ingredients in a blender and process until smooth.

BERRY SMOOTHIE

Ingredients:
- 1 cup frozen blueberries or 1 cup fresh blueberries
- 15 oz coconut milk
- Stevia to taste
- 1 scoop of hemp protein
- 1 teaspoon cinnamon (optional)

Instructions:
- Place all ingredients into a blender. Blend until mixed thoroughly.
- Serve right away.

COCONUT BERRY SMOOTHIE

Ingredients:
- 1 Cup Frozen Blackberries
- 1 Frozen Banana
- 1 Teaspoon Chia Seeds
- 1 Inch Piece of Fresh Ginger
- 1 Cup Coconut Milk
- 1 scoop of HEMP protein
- 2 Tablespoons Toasted Coconut

Instructions:
- Combine all the ingredients in a blender and process until smooth.

VANILLA HOT DRINK

Ingredients:

- 3 cups unsweetened almond milk
- Stevia to taste
- 1 scoop of hemp protein
- 1/2 Tbsp. ground cinnamon (or more to taste)
- 1/2 Tbsp. vanilla extract

Instructions:

- Place the almond milk into a pitcher. Place ground cinnamon, hemp, vanilla extract in a small saucepan over medium high heat. Heat until the pure liquid stevia is just melted and then pour the pure liquid stevia mixture into the pitcher.

- Stir until the pure liquid stevia is well combined with the almond milk. Place the pitcher in the fridge and allow it to chill for at least two hours. Stir well before serving.

ALMOND BUTTER SMOOTHIES

Ingredients:

- 1 scoop of hemp protein
- 1 tbsp almond butter
- 1 cup of hemp milk
- 1 banana, preferably frozen
- few ice cubes

Instructions:

- Blend all ingredients together and enjoy!

CHOCO WALNUT DELIGHT

Ingredients:
- 1 scoop Hemp Protein
- 1 oz dark sugar free chocolate broken up.
- 2 tbsp walnuts chopped/crushed
- 1 cup hemp milk or nut milk alternative
- Handful of ice cubes

Instructions:
- Blend everything together in a strong blender until thoroughly processed.

RASPBERRY HEMP SMOOTHIE

Ingredients:
- 1 cup hemp milk or milk alternative
- 1/2 cup raspberries (fresh or frozen)
- 2 tablespoons hemp protein powder
- Stevia to taste
- 3 to 4 ice cubes

Instructions:
- Add ingredients to a blender and blend until smooth.

CHOCO BANANA SMOOTHIE

Ingredients:
- 1 cup milk or milk alternative
- 2 peeled frozen bananas
- ice cubes
- 2 tablespoons hulled hemp seed
- 2 tablespoons hemp protein powder
- 1 tablespoons organic cocoa powder
- 5-7 drops liquid stevia to sweeten
- 1/4 teaspoon cinnamon
- 1/4 teaspoon vanilla

Instructions:
- Put all ingredients into a blender. Blend until smooth.

BLUEBERRY ALMOND SMOOTHIE

Ingredients:
- 1 cup almond milk
- 1 cup frozen unsweetened blueberries
- 1 Tbsp cold-pressed organic flaxseed oil
- 1 tbsp hemp protein powder

Instructions:
- Combine milk and blueberries in a blender, and blend for 1 minute.
- Transfer to glass, and stir in flaxseed oil.

HAZELNUT BUTTER AND BANANA SMOOTHIE

Ingredients:
- 1 cup nut milk
- 1 cup hemp milk
- 1 Tbsp creamy natural unsalted hazelnut butter
- 1 ripe banana
- stevia drops to taste
- ice cubes
- 1 tbsp hemp protein powder

Instructions:
- Combine ingredients in a blender. Process until smooth. Pour into a tall glass and serve.

VANILLA BLUEBERRY SMOOTHIE

Ingredients:
- 2 cups hemp milk
- 1 c fresh blueberries
- Handful of ice OR 1 cup frozen blueberries
- 1 Tbsp flaxseed oil
- 1 tbsp hemp protein powder

Instructions:
- Combine milk, and fresh blueberries plus ice (or frozen blueberries) in a blender. Blend for 1 minute, transfer to a glass, and stir in flaxseed oil.

CHOCOLATE RASPBERRY SMOOTHIE

Ingredients:
- 1 cup almond milk
- 1 cup chocolate chips-sugar free
- 1 cup fresh raspberries
- 1 tsp hemp protein powder
- Handful of ice OR 1 cup frozen raspberries

Instructions:
- Combine ingredients in a blender and blend.

PEACH SMOOTHIE

Ingredients:
- 1 cup hemp milk
- 1 c frozen unsweetened peaches
- 1 tsp cold-pressed organic flaxseed oil
- 1 tsp hemp protein powder

Instructions:
- Place milk and frozen, unsweetened peaches in a blender and blend for 1 minute. Transfer to glass, and stir in flaxseed oil.

ZESTY CITRUS SMOOTHIE

Ingredients:
- 1 cup almond milk
- 1/2 cup lemon juice
- 1 orange peeled, and sliced into sections
- Handful of ice
- 1 Tbsp flaxseed oil
- 1 tsp hemp protein powder

Instructions:
- Combine milk, lemon juice, orange, and ice in a blender. Blend for 1 minute, transfer to a glass, and stir in flaxseed oil.

APPLE SMOOTHIE

Ingredients:
- 1 cup hemp milk
- 1 cup hemp milk
- 1 tsp apple pie spice
- 1 apple peeled and chopped
- 1 Tbsp cashew butter
- Handful of ice
- 1 tbsp hemp protein powder

Instructions:
- Combine ingredients in a blender. Blend for 1 minute, transfer to a glass, and eat with a spoon.

PINEAPPLE SMOOTHIE

Ingredients:
- 1 cup almond milk
- 1 oz fresh pineapple
- Handful of ice
- 1 tbsp hemp protein powder
- 1 Tbsp cold-pressed organic flaxseed oil

Instructions:
- Place milk, canned pineapple in a blender, add ice, and whip for 1 minute. Transfer to glass and stir in flaxseed oil.

STRAWBERRY SMOOTHIE

Ingredients:
- 1 cup almond milk
- 1 cup frozen, unsweetened strawberries
- 1 tbsp hemp protein powder
- 1 tsp flaxseed oil

Instructions:
- Combine milk and strawberries in a blender. Blend, transfer to glass, and stir in flaxseed oil.

PINEAPPLE COCONUT SMOOTHIE

Ingredients:
- 1 Cup pineapple chunks
- 1 Cup coconut milk
- 1/2 Cup pineapple juice

- 1 ripe banana
- 1/2 - 3/4 Cup ice cubes
- Pure liquid stevia to taste
- 1 tbsp hemp protein powder

Instructions:

- In a blender, combine the pineapple chunks, coconut milk, banana, ice and pure liquid stevia. Puree until smooth.

VANILLA SMOOTHIE

Ingredients:

- 1 cup almond milk
- 1 cup almond butter
- 1 tsp vanilla extract
- 2 cups ice
- Stevia vanilla liquid to taste
- 1 tbsp Vanilla Protein Powder

Instructions:

- Add all ingredients except ice to the blender. Puree well. Add ice and blend until ice is all crushed and smoothie is well blended and smooth.

COCO ORANGE DELISH SMOOTHIE

Ingredients:

- 1/2 cup fresh squeezed orange juice
- 1 tablespoon hemp protein powder
- 1/2 cup full fat coconut milk from the can
- 1 teaspoon vanilla

- 1/2 -1 cup crushed ice

Instructions:

- Add all ingredients to a blender. Blend until smooth and add ice as needed to get the consistency you like.

BABY KALE PINEAPPLE SMOOTHIE

Ingredients:
- 1 cup almond milk
- 1/2 cup frozen pineapple
- 1 cup Kale
- 1 tablespoon hemp protein powder

Instructions:

- Place the almond milk, pineapple, and greens in the blender and blend until smooth.

STRAWBERRY COCONUT SMOOTHIE

Ingredients:
- cup coconut milk
- frozen banana, sliced
- cups frozen strawberries
- 1 teaspoon vanilla extract
- 1 tablespoon hemp protein powder

Instructions:

- Add all ingredients to the blender and blend until smooth.

BLUEBERRY BONANZA SMOOTHIES

Ingredients:
- 1/4 cup canned coconut or almond milk
- 1/2 cup water
- 1 medium banana, sliced
- 1 cup frozen blueberries
- 1 tablespoon raw almonds

Instructions:
- Add the ingredients to a blender. Blend until smooth. Serve.

EPACH COCONUT SMOOTHIE

Ingredients:
- 1 cup full fat coconut milk, chilled
- 1 cup ice
- large fresh peaches, peeled and cut into chunks
- Fresh lemon zest, to taste
- 1 tablespoon hemp protein powder

Instructions:
- Add coconut milk, ice and peaches blender. Using a zester, add a few gratings of fresh lemon zest. Blend on high speed until smooth.

KEY LIME PIE SMOOTHIE

Ingredients:
- 1 cup coconut milk
- 1 cup ice
- 1/2 avocado
- zest and juice of 2 limes

- Pure liquid stevia to taste
- 1 tablespoon hemp protein powder

Instructions:

- Add all ingredients to a blender and blend until smooth.

HIGH PROTEIN AND NUTRITIONAL SMOOTHIE

Ingredients:

- 1 cup almond milk
- 1/2 Avocado
- Strawberries
- 1/2 Bananas
- 1/2 cup Raw Kale or spinach
- 1/4 cup Carrot Juice, water can be used
- 1 cup Coconut Yogurt..or almond milk
- 1 tablespoon hemp protein powder

Instructions:

- Add everything to your blender, and blend to your preferred consistency . ; more water or ice can be added to help with your preferred texture/thickness.

PINEAPPLE PROTEIN SMOOTHIE

Ingredients:
- 1 cup pineapple chunks
- 1 cup coconut milk
- 1 banana
- 1 cup ice cubes
- 1 tsp vanilla bean powder
- pinch low sodium salt
- 1 tablespoon hemp protein powder

Instructions:
- Put everything into a high speed blender and blend until smooth.

RASPBERRY COCONUT SMOOTHIE

Ingredients:
- 1 cup coconut milk
- medium banana, peeled sliced and frozen
- 2 teaspoons coconut extract (optional)
- 1 cup frozen raspberries
- 1 tablespoon hemp protein powder

Instructions:
- Add coconut milk, frozen banana slices and coconut extract to your blender. Pulse 1-2 minutes until smooth.
- Add frozen raspberries and continue to pulse until smooth.

GINGER CARROT PROTEIN SMOOTHIE

Ingredients:

- 3/4 cup carrot juice
- 1 tablespoon hemp protein powder
- 1 tablespoon hulled hemp seeds
- 1/2 apple
- 3 to 4 ice cubes
- 1/2 inch piece fresh ginger

Instructions:

- Add to a blender and blend until smooth.

GREEN SMOOTHIE

Ingredients:

- 1 carrot
- 3 cups spinach
- 2 small tomatoes
- 3/4 to 1 cup of water
- 1 apple
- 1 cup strawberry
- 1/3 avocado

Instructions:

- Add all the ingredients to your blender last. Blend on high for 30 seconds or until the smoothie is creamy.

GREENS SMOOTHIE WITH MANGO AND LIME

Ingredients:
- 2 tablespoons fresh lime juice
- 2 cups stemmed and chopped collard greens or spinach
- 1 1/2 cups frozen mango
- 1 cup green grapes

Directions:
- Combine the lime juice, cup water, the collard greens, mango, and grapes in a blender and puree until smooth, about 1 minute, adding more water to reach the desired consistency.

SUMPTIONS SPINACH SMOOTHIE WITH AVOCADO

Ingredients:
- 2 cups apple juice
- 2 cups stemmed and chopped spinach or kale
- 1 apple-unpeeled, cored, and chopped
- 1 avocado, chopped

Directions:
- Combine the apple juice, spinach, apple, and avocado in a blender and puree until smooth, about 1 minute, adding water to reach the desired consistency.

KALE SMOOTHIE WITH PINEAPPLE

Ingredients:
- 1 cup coconut milk
- 2 cups stemmed and chopped kale or spinach
- 1 cup chopped pineapple

1 ripe banana, chopped

Directions:
- Combine the coconut milk, cup water, the kale, pineapple, and banana in a blender and puree until smooth, about 1 minute, adding more water to reach the desired consistency.

KINKY KALE-APPLE SMOOTHIE

Ingredients:
- 1 cup chopped kale, ribs and thick stems removed
- 1 small stalk celery, chopped
- 1 banana
- 1 cup apple juice
- 1 cup ice

- 1 tablespoon fresh lemon juice

Directions:

- Place the kale, celery, banana, apple juice, ice, and lemon juice in a blender. Blend until smooth and frothy.

PEAR GREEN PROTEIN

Ingredients:
- 2 scoops Protein vanilla
- 1 cup unsweetened almond milk
- 1 cup spinach
- 1 pear, cored
- 1/2 teaspoon of matcha tea powder

Directions:
- Combine all ingredients in a blender and mix until smooth.

ORANGE KALE SMOOTHIE

Ingredients:
- 2 scoops Protein vanilla
- 1 cup water
- 1 cup raw chopped kale
- 1 orange, peel and seeds removed
- 1/2 teaspoon of spirulina powder
- 1 pinch of ground cinnamon
- 1 pinch of ginger powder

Directions:
- Combine all ingredients in a blender and mix until smooth.

GINGER-ORANGE GREEN SMOOTHIE

Ingredients:
- 2 cups filtered water
- generous handfuls fresh spinach
- romaine leaves (optional)
- 2 navel oranges
- 2 ripe bananas
- 1"-2" knob of fresh ginger
- 1 cucumber (optional) peel if not organic

Directions:
- Rinse and prep veggies.

- If you have a high-powered blender, throw everything in and blend until smooth. If not, first blend the spinach and romaine until smooth, then add the remaining ingredients and blend.

BLUEBERRY MINT SMOOTHIE
Ingredients:

- 2 cups spinach
- 2 cups blueberry
- 1 kiwi
- 3-4 large mint leaves
- 1 cup coconut water
- 1 cup ice

Instructions:
- Put all ingredients in a blender and mix it up!

SPRING DETOX

Ingredients:
- 1 cup green tea, chilled
- 1 cup loosely packed cilantro
- 1 cup loosely packed organic baby kale (or another baby green)
- 1 cup cucumber
- 1 cup pineapple
- juice of 1 lemon
- 1 tablespoon fresh ginger, grated
- 1 avocado

Instructions:
- Place ingredients into a blender and puree until smooth.

GORGEOUS GREEN

Ingredients:
- 3/4 cup milk

- 2 big handfuls spinach
- 1/2 banana
- 1/4 cup raw rolled oats
- 1/2 scoop chocolate protein powder
- 1 tbsp flax
- Granola topping

Directions:

- Place ingredients into a blender and puree until smooth.

SWEET MELON

Ingredients:

- 1/2 honeydew melon, cut into chunks
- 1/2 cup light coconut milk
- 1-2 leaves fresh mint (plus more for garnish)
- 1/2-1 tsp. fresh lime juice
- 1 cup ice
- Drizzle of honey or coconut nectar, to taste (optional, depending on how sweet your melon is)

Directions:

- Cut your melon in half, remove the seeds, and slice away the outer rind.

- Cut the melon into chunks, and add to your blender along with the coconut milk, mint, lime, and ice.

- Blend until smooth. Taste, and adjust sweetness

with honey or coconut nectar. Serve with a garnish of mint, or fresh melon slices.

PEACHY GREEN

Ingredients:
- 1 cup unsweetened almond milk
- 1 cup frozen peaches
- 1/2 cup frozen pineapple
- 1/2 banana
- 2 cups kale
- 1 tablespoon ground flaxseed

Instructions:
- Add all ingredients to the blender. Mix until smooth.

KALE PINA

Ingredients:
- 2/3 cup unsweetened vanilla almond milk
- 2 hand-fulls kale
- 1/3 cup pineapple chunks
- 1/2 ripe avocado
- 1 scoop protein powder
- 1 cup ice cubes

Instructions:
- Put all ingredients into a blender and puree until smooth!

ALMOND PEANUT SMOOTHIE

Ingredients:
- 3/4 cup almond milk
- 1/4 cup strong espresso, slightly cooled
- 1/2 cup frozen banana
- 1/4 cup smooth peanut butter
- 1/4 cup dark chocolate, roughly chopped
- ice, as needed
- agave syrup, optional to sweeten

Directions:
- Pour milk and espresso into a blender jar. Add frozen banana and peanut butter. Add about a half a cup of ice. Cover with lid and press the auto smoothie button.

ENERGY SMOOTHIE

Ingredients:
- 2 cups romaine lettuce or baby spinach
- 1 cups tomato
- 1 cup coconut water or filtered water
- 1 cup chopped carrot
- 1 whole cucumber
- 1 avocado
- 1 whole lime peeled
- 2 garlic cloves
- 1 tsp sea salt

Instructions:

• Put all of the ingredients in your blender and puree until smooth and creamy.

THE DETOX DELIGHT

Ingredients:
- 1/4 cup filtered water
- 1 red apples, diced
- 1 cup baby spinach
- 1" piece of fresh ginger, peeled and diced
- 1 teaspoon flax oil (optional)
- 1/2 teaspoon wheat grass powder (optional)
- tiny pinch cayenne pepper (optional)
- 1 cup ice cubes

Directions:
• Throw all of the ingredients into your high-speed blender and blast for 30 to 60 seconds until well combined.

PUMPKIN PIE DRINK

Ingredients:
- 2 cups filtered water
- 1/2 cup raw, unsalted cashews, soaked
- 1/4 cup rolled oats
- 1 cup canned or freshly mashed pumpkin
- 1 fresh or frozen ripe banana
- 2 tablespoons maple syrup, plus or more to taste
- 1 teaspoon natural vanilla extract
- 1 1/4 teaspoons ground cinnamon, plus more to taste
- 1/2 teaspoon ground ginger, plus more to taste
- 1/4 teaspoon ground nutmeg, plus more to taste
- pinch ground cloves
- pinch of Celtic sea salt
- cup ice cubes

Directions:
- Throw all the ingredients (except the ice into the blender and blast on high for 30 to 60 seconds until smooth and creamy.

- Add the ice and blast again for about 10 seconds until chilled.

ROSE MELON JUICE

Ingredients:

- 2 cups chopped seedless watermelon, chilled
- 1 teaspoon finely grated lemon zest
- 1 lemon, peeled and seeded
- 1/2 teaspoons finely chopped rosemary
- 1/2 cup frozen pineapple
- 1/4 cup frozen strawberries
- 3 drops liquid stevia, plus more to taste (optional)

Directions:

- Throw all of the ingredients into your blender and blast on high for 30 to 60 seconds, until well combined.

CARROT PECAN JUICE

Ingredients:

- 2 cups filtered water
- 1/4 cups soaked raw pecans
- 2 medium o carrots - tops removed, peeled, and chopped
- 1/2 teaspoons ground cinnamon
- 1 crushed cardamom pod or 1/4 teaspoon cardamom powder
- 2 teaspoons vanilla extract
- 2 tablespoons maple syrup

Instructions:

- Throw all of the ingredients into your blender and

blast on high until smooth and creamy. Strain with a nut milk bag or fine mesh sieve to remove the pulp.

WINTER WONDERLAND

Ingredients:
- 1/2 cup frozen blueberries
- 1/2 avocado
- 1/2 small frozen banana
- handful baby spinach (or kale)
- 2 cups water
- 1 tbsp cocoa powder
- 1 tbsp raw honey
- Pinch of cayenne

Directions:
- Throw all of the ingredients into your high-speed blender and blast for 30 to 60 seconds until well combined.

CARROT CINNAMON SMOOTHIE

Ingredients:

- 2 medium carrots, peeled and chopped
- 1/2 frozen banana
- 2 cups spinach
- 1 cup unsweetened soy milk
- 1/2 scoop vanilla protein powder
- 1/8 cup golden raisins
- 1/2 teaspoon cinnamon
- Dash of ground nutmeg
- Dash of ground cloves

ice cubes

Directions:

- Throw all of the ingredients into your high-speed blender and blast for 30 to 60 seconds until well combined.

- Enjoy right away while still fresh, and give a little stir if separation occurs.

ARTHRITIS ASSISTANCE

Ingredients:

- Peeled and cut fresh pineapple chunks of one medium size pineapple
- 1 green cardamom
- 1 inch fresh ginger (peeled and cut)

Directions:

- Blend or juice all the above in a slow juicer and enjoy a different flavor and taste.

SKINNY CRUISER

Ingredients:

- 8 celery stalks
- 2 medium cucumbers
- 1 bunch parsley
- 1 small lemon

Directions:

- Throw all of the ingredients into your high-speed blender and blast for 30 to 60 seconds until well combined.

- Enjoy right away while still fresh, and give a little stir if separation occurs.

LIVER DETOX JUICE

Ingredients:

- 1 stalk Celery
- 1 carrot
- 1 apple
- handful dandelion
- handful parsley
- 1 red cabbage
- fresh ginger root

Directions:

- Throw all of the ingredients into your high-speed blender and blast for 30 to 60 seconds until well combined.

- Pour some Aloe Vera Juice in the jar then add the obtained juice.

HORMONE HELPER

Ingredients

- 1 aloe vera leaf
- 1 cucumber
- 4 stalks of kale
- 1 onion
- 2 carrots

Directions:

- Throw all of the ingredients into your high-speed

blender and blast for 30 to 60 seconds until well combined.

- Enjoy right away while still fresh, and give a little stir if separation occurs.

GRAPEFRUITS BEET JUICE

Ingredients:

- 2-3 golden beet roots (no leaves)
- 6 carrots
- 1 large pink grapefruit
- 1 green apple
- 2" ginger root
- 1 lemon, no peel

Directions:

- Throw all of the ingredients into your high-speed blender and blast for 30 to 60 seconds until well combined.

- Enjoy right away while still fresh, and give a little stir if separation occurs.

BETTER BEET JUICE

Ingredients :
- 1 beetroot
- 4 to 5 carrots
- 3 to 4 celery stalks
- Handful of cilantro
- lime, with peel
- 1" chunk of fresh ginger root, or more to taste

Directions:
- Throw all of the ingredients into your high-speed blender and blast for 30 to 60 seconds until well combined.

- Enjoy right away while still fresh, and give a little stir if separation occurs.

WINTER JUICE

Ingredients:
- 6 carrots
- 6 stalks of celery
- 1 beetroot
- Handful of parsley
- 1 bunch of kale
- 1" chunk of fresh ginger root, or more to taste

Directions:
- Throw all of the ingredients into your high-speed blender and blast for 30 to 60 seconds until well

combined.

- Enjoy right away while still fresh, and give a little stir if separation occurs.

VEGGIES JUICE

Ingredients:
- Baby cucumbers
- Tomatoes
- Bitter melon

Directions:
- Extract the juice of the above three, through a slow juice.

BROCCOLI JUICE

Ingredients:
- 1 head of broccoli
- 2 carrots
- 2 handfuls of spinach
- 1 red apple

Instructions:
- Throw all of the ingredients into your high-speed blender and blast for 30 to 60 seconds until well combined.
- Enjoy right away while still fresh.

AMAZING APPLE FLAVOR

Ingredients:

- A bunch of Kale
- A bunch of Spinach
- 1 Celery stalk
- 1 Fuji apple
- 1 tablespoon chia seeds (optional)

Directions:

- Throw all of the ingredients into your high-speed blender and blast for 30 to 60 seconds until well combined.
- Enjoy right away while still fresh, and give a little stir if separation occurs.
- Stir in the chia seeds to thicken up the juice and make a more sustaining snack or meal out of it.

Peach & Funnel Drink

Ingredients:

- 1 head iceberg lettuce
- 1/2 head green cabbage
- 1 inch square of fennel bulb (be generous)
- 2 inches ginger root (again, be generous)
- 2 peaches (remove the pit!)
- 10 grapes-green

Directions:

- Throw all of the ingredients into your high-speed blender and blast for 30 to 60 seconds until well combined.

SUNSET SENSATION

Ingredients

- 1 Large Celery Stalks
- 2 Large Carrots
- 1 Pear
- 1 Medium Apple
- 1 Lemon Peel On
- 1/4 Honeydew Lemon
- 1/4 Small Pineapple
- 1" Root Ginger (optional)

Directions:

- Throw all of the ingredients into your high-speed blender and blast for 30 to 60 seconds until well combined.

- Enjoy right away while still fresh, and give a little stir if separation occurs.

SPICY VEGGIE

Ingredients:

- 2 large juicy tomatoes
- 2 carrots
- 1 large red chili
- 1 handful of coriander (also known as cilantro) leaves and stalks

Directions:

- Juice all of the above ingredients and then give the juice a good stir.

COOL CUCUMBER KIWI

Ingredients
- 2 Kiwis
- 1/2 Cucumber
- 5 Strawberries
- 1 Celery Rib
- 2-3 Kale Leaves
- Handful of Dandelion greens or Spinach
- 1 Apple
- 1 Carrot

Directions
- Throw all of the ingredients into your high-speed blender and blast for 30 to 60 seconds until well combined.

- Enjoy right away while still fresh, and give a little stir if separation occurs.

PARSNIP-KALE-TOMATO

Ingredients:
- 10 Kale Leaves
- 2 Parsnips
- 1 Tomato
- 2 Celery Stalks
- 1 Apple (or more for desired sweetness)

Instructions:
- Throw all of the ingredients into your high-speed blender and blast for 30 to 60 seconds until

well combined.

- Enjoy right away while still fresh, and give a little stir if separation occurs.

FABULOUS FRUITY

Ingredients:
- 2 apples
- 2 pears
- 1 kiwi fruit
- 2 oranges
- 1 lemon
- A handful of mint leaves

Instructions:
- Transfer to a blender with 1/2 cup of water.

FRUITY FAST

Ingredients:
- 1 Red Apple
- 1 Pear
- 2 Carrots
- 1/2 Papaya
- 1 Bunch Spinach
- 1 Blood Orange

Instructions:

- Transfer to blender with 1/2 cup of water

CELERY & CUCUMBER JUICE

Ingredients:
- 1/2 cucumber
- 2 sticks of celery
- 1 orange
- 1 handful of baby spinach
- 1/2 green bell pepper
- 10 leaves of kale
- 1 tomato
- 2 carrots

Instructions:
- Throw all of the ingredients into your high-speed blender and blast for 30 to 60 seconds until well combined.

- Enjoy right away while still fresh, and give a little stir if separation occurs.

HOT AND SPICY JUICE

Ingredients:
- 1 Large bunch Kale (10-12 leaves)
- 1 Small Beet plus greens
- 1 Medium Watermelon Radish
- 2 hot peppers (or to taste)

- 2 large cucumbers
- 1 head of celery (5-6 stalks)
- 2 apples
- 1 clove garlic
- 1 shallot or 2 scallions
- 1/2 cup cilantro
- 1 whole lemon
- 1 whole lime
- 5-8 ripe tomatoes
- 1 inch of ginger (optional)

Instructions:

Throw all of the ingredients into your high-speed blender and blast until well combined.

GORGEOUS GREENS

Ingredients:

- 10 stalks kale
- 1 apple
- A handful spinach
- 1 pear
- 2 stalks celery

Instructions:

- Juice all the ingredients in a juice extractor.
- Juice kale & spinach between fruits

CINNAMON COCONUT SMOOTHIE

Ingredients:

- 1/2 Cup Coconut Milk
- 1 Large Egg Yolks
- 1 Medium Banana
- 1/4 Cup Ice
- 1/2 tsp Cinnamon

Instructions:

- Throw all of the ingredients into your high-speed blender and blast for 30 to 60 seconds until well combined.

- Enjoy right away while still fresh, and give a little stir if separation occurs.

BLUEBERRY AVOCADO SMOOTHIE

Ingredients:

- 1 Cup Water
- 1 Tbsp Avocado
- 1 Cup Blueberries, Frozen
- 2 Cups Spinach

Instructions:

- Throw all of the ingredients into your high-speed blender and blast for 30 to 60 seconds until well combined.

- Enjoy right away while still fresh, and give a little stir if separation occurs.

BANANA RADISH DRINK

Ingredients
- 1 Cup of Water
- 1 Medium Banana
- 10 Large Radish, Sliced
- 1 Cup of Ice

Instructions:
- Throw all of the ingredients into your high-speed blender and blast for 30 to 60 seconds until well combined.

- Enjoy right away while still fresh, and give a little stir if separation occurs.

ROASTED CAULIFLOWER AND SWEET POTATO SOUP

Ingredients
- 1 head of cauliflower, chopped into florets
- 1 medium-sized sweet potatoes, peeled and cubed;
- 2 garlic cloves, peeled;
- 1 tsp. paprika
- 5 cups vegetable or chicken stock;
- 1/2 cup coconut or almond milk;
- 1 tbsp. olive oil;
- Sea salt and freshly ground black pepper;

Instructions
- Preheat your oven to 400 F.

- Place the cauliflower florets, cubed potatoes, and

garlic on a baking sheet.Drizzle with olive oil, and season to taste with salt and pepper.

- Roast in the oven for 35 to 40 minutes or until the vegetables are soft.Transfer the vegetables from the baking sheet to a saucepan.

- Pour the vegetable stock into the saucepan, and add the paprika. Bring to a simmer and puree the soup using an immersion blender.

- Pour in the coconut or almond milk, and give everything a good stir. Continue simmering until warm, and season to taste before serving.

TURKEY AND VEGETABLE SOUP

Ingredients
- 2 cups leftover turkey, chopped;
- 1 onion, diced;
- 3 to 4 carrots, diced;
- 2 parsnips, diced;
- 2 celery stalks, diced;
- 1 cup cauliflower, riced;
- 2 cups cabbage, shredded;
- 2 bay leaves;
- 2 garlic cloves, minced;
- 1 tsp. ground sage;
- 1 tsp. thyme;

- Sea salt and freshly ground black pepper to taste

Turkey stock

- turkey carcass or 5 lbs. turkey parts (preferably bony parts, like necks and backs);
- 2 yellow onions, quartered;
- 2 celery ribs, cut into big chunks;
- 2 carrots, cut into big chunks;
- 3 garlic cloves;
- 2 sprigs fresh thyme;
- 1 bay leaf;
- 2 quarts cold water
- Freshly ground black pepper

Instructions:

- Place the turkey carcass or parts in a saucepan, add all the remaining ingredients for the stock, and season to taste with pepper.

- Fill the saucepan with water and bring to a boil. Lower heat to a light simmer, and simmer for 4 to 8 hours. (adding water if necessary).

- Strain the stock with a fine mesh sieve, throwing away all the remaining ingredients. Set aside .

- Pick through the carcass. Remove any meat you find, and add it to the meat for the soup.

- Add all the ingredients for the soup in a large saucepan. Fill the pan with the turkey stock, and season to taste. Bring to a simmer, and simmer for 45 minutes to 1 hour.

CREAM OF CHICKEN AND LEEK SOUP

Ingredients

- 1 medium leek, sliced;
- 3 cups cooked chicken, diced;
- 2 cloves garlic, minced;
- 1 tbsp. tapioca starch;
- 4 cups chicken stock;
- 1 cup water;
- 1 cup coconut milk;
- 1 tbsp olive oil
- Sea salt and freshly ground black pepper;

Instructions:

- Melt some cooking fat in a large saucepan placed over a medium-high heat. Add the leeks to the saucepan and cook until soft, about 10 minutes.

- Season to taste with salt and pepper. Add the chicken stock and water and bring to a boil while stirring. Lower the heat and let simmer for about 15 minutes.

- Add the chicken and coconut milk and cook until the whole soup is warmed through. Remove one ladle of warm broth from the soup.

- Mix it with the tapioca starch in a small bowl, and then slowly add the mixture back to the soup while stirring, until the soup reaches your desired consistency. Adjust the seasoning and serve.

WILD MUSHROOM SOUP

Ingredients

- 1 lb. mixed wild mushrooms, sliced;
- 1 large shallots, diced;
- 1 tbsp. fresh thyme;
- 2 cups chicken stock;
- 1 cup. coconut milk;
- 1 tbsp. ghee;
- 1 cup parsley, chopped;
- 1 tbsp. tapioca starch; (optional)
- Sea salt and freshly ground pepper;

Instructions:

- Melt the ghee in a large saucepan placed over medium high. Add the shallots and saute for 3 to 4 minutes.

- Add the mushrooms and thyme and cook for about 8 minutes. Add the chicken stock and bring to a boil. Turn down the heat to medium- low, and let simmer for 15 minutes.

- Stir in the coconut milk, season to taste, and let simmer for another 5 minutes.

- Stir in the tapioca starch if you like your soups thicker. Mix in the chopped parsley and serve.

OLD FASHIONED CABBAGE SOUP

Ingredients
- 2 chicken breasts, cut into chunks
- 1 leek, sliced
- 2 carrots, sliced
- 2 celery stalks, sliced
- 2 sweet potatoes, diced
- 3 cups shredded cabbage
- 1 cup rutabaga, diced
- 6 cups chicken stock
- 2 garlic cloves, minced
- Sea salt and freshly ground black pepper
- 1 tbsp olive oil

Instructions:
- Melt some cooking fat in a large saucepan placed over a medium-high heat. Add the chicken and garlic and cook for 4 to 5 minutes.

- Add the carrots, celery, and leek, and cook for another 4 minutes. Incorporate all the remaining ingredients, season to taste, and give everything a good stir.

- Cover the soup and cook for 15 to 20 minutes, or until the vegetables are soft.

ROASTED TASTY TOMATO SOUP

Ingredients:
- 1 lb fresh tomatoes
- 1 red onion, medium
- 1 small head garlic, peeled
- 1 tbsp olive oil
- 1 tsp low sodium salt
- 1/2 tsp fresh cracked black pepper
- 1 tsp oregano
- 3/4 cup low sodium chicken broth
- 15 oz tomato sauce, canned

Instructions:
- Preheat the oven to 375 degrees F. Cube tomatoes and onion. Place on a baking sheet. Drizzle with olive oil and sprinkle with seasonings. Slice butter into small pieces on top of vegetables.

- Roast for 30 minutes, stirring halfway after 15 minutes. Allow roasted vegetables to cool for 10 minutes. Puree vegetables, broth and tomato sauce in a blender until smooth, scraping down the sides several times while blending.

- Heat tomato soup in a saucepan allowing the soup to slowly simmer for a few minutes to blend the flavors together. Serve hot topped with chives.

THAI COCONUT TURKEY SOUP

Ingredients:
- A small splash of oil
- 1 onion, sliced thin
- A big handful of shiitake mushrooms, cut in half
- 2 cloves of garlic, finely minced
- 1 inch piece of ginger, julienned
- A handful of cherry tomatoes
- 2 cups turkey stock
- 1 cup shredded cooked turkey
- 1 cup canned coconut milk
- low sodium salt to taste
- A small handful of cilantro

Instructions:
- Stir fry onion, garlic, ginger and then add mushrooms and tomatoes.

- Add turkey meat and fry for a few minutes till slightly browned. Add stock and simmer for 20 minutes.

- Serve warm and sprinkle chives on top.

HEARTY CHICKEN SOUP

Ingredients:

- 1 large chicken breasts, skin removed and cut into inch strips
- 28 oz can of diced tomatoes
- 32 ounces low sodium organic chicken broth
- 1 sweet onion, diced
- 2 cups of shredded carrots
- 2 cups chopped celery
- 1 bunch of cilantro chopped fine
- 3 cloves of garlic, minced
- 1 Tbsp tomato paste
- 1 tsp chili powder
- 1 tsp cumin
- l salt & pepper to taste
- 1 tbsp olive oil
- 1-2 cups water

Instructions:

- In a crockpot place a dash of olive oil and about 1 cup chicken broth. Add onions, garlic, jalapeno, low sodium salt and pepper and cook until soft, adding more broth as needed.

- Then add all of your remaining ingredients and enough water to fill the top of your pot. Cover and let cook on low for about 2 hrs, adjusting low sodium salt & pepper as needed.

- Once the chicken is fully cooked, you should be

able to shred it very easily. I simply used the back of a wooden spoon and pressed the cooked chicken against the side of the pot.

- Top with avocado slices and fresh cilantro. Enjoy!

TRIPLE SQUASH SOUP

Ingredients:

- 1 butternut squash
- 1 gold acorn squash
- 1 white acorn squash
- 1-2 cups vegetable stock (depending on squash size, and how thick you want the soup)
- 3 cups diced turkey breast
- 1/4 cup light coconut milk
- 1 tbsp. olive oil
- low sodium salt for seasoning

Instructions:

- Preheat the oven to 400 degrees. Halve each squash, scoop out the seeds (and save them for toasting), and then slice into 1-1 1/2 inch thick crescents.

- Spread the squash on an aluminum foil-lined baking sheet and coat lightly with the olive oil. Season with low sodium salt. Roast for about 30 minutes, or until golden brown (turning once midway through baking).

- When the squash has cooled from the oven slightly, spoon off the meat from the skin.

- In a medium to large pot, bring the turkey meat, the meat of all the squash and 1 1/2 cups of vegetable stock to a boil. Turn the heat to low and stir in the coconut milk.

- Remove from heat to puree the soup. You can use an immersion blender, or transfer everything to a traditional blender.

- Blend until smooth, adding any additional stock to achieve the consistency you like.

GINGER CARROT SOUP

Ingredients:

- 1 tbsp unsalted butter or coconut oil
- 1/2 pounds carrots (6-7 large carrots), sliced
- 2 cups chopped white or yellow onion
- 1 cup diced turkey breast
- low sodium salt
- 2 teaspoons minced ginger
- 4 cups low sodium chicken stock
- 2 cups water
- 1 large strips of zest from an orange

Instructions:

- Heat up the butter or coconut oil in a large soup pot. Add the chopped carrots, turkey breast and onion to the pot and cook over medium heat for 5-10 minutes. Add in the remaining ingredients (ginger, orange zest, water, and stock).

- The orange zest will be pulled out prior to pureeing so make sure they are in large, easy to identify strips rather than small pieces.

- Bring to a boil for 10 minutes. Remove orange zest strips. Puree the mixture with an immersion blender.

WATERCRESS SOUP

Ingredients:
- 1 quart low sodium chicken stock
- 1 medium leek
- 1 bunch watercress
- 1 large onion
- 1 cup celeriac root skinned and chopped
- 2 cups diced chicken breast
- salt and pepper to taste

Instructions:
- Gently heat the chicken stock in the pot. In the fry pan saute the onion, leek and celeriac until soft.

- Place the onion, leek, chicken and celeriac in the pot of stock reserving 1/3 aside.

- Season with low sodium salt and pepper. Add the bunch of watercress and simmer a few minutes until it is wilted.

- With the immersion blender, blend the soup. Add

the chopped vegetables that you reserved, back into the pot.

CURRIED BUTTERNUT SOUP

Ingredients:

- 1 medium butternut squash, cut in half lengthwise, seeds removed
- 1 cup diced chicken breast
- 1 medium yellow onion, chopped
- 1 inch piece fresh ginger, peeled and diced or grated
- 1 tablespoon curry powder
- 1 can coconut milk
- 1 1/2 Cups chicken broth
- 1 tbspCoconut Oil
- low sodium salt and pepper

Instructions:

- Preheat the oven to 425 degrees. Melt a tablespoon of coconut oil in a roasting pan.

- Place squash, cut side down in a roasting pan. Roast 45 minutes to an hour, or until fork tender.

- Add ginger and curry powder and saute 2 more minutes.Scoop flesh out of roasted squash and add to apple mixture.

- Add coconut milk, chicken and chicken broth. Stir to incorporate ingredients and bring to a boil.

- Simmer mixture, uncovered for 20 minutes. Using either a high power mixer or an immersion blender, blend soup until it's smooth.

CELERY CASHEW CREAM SOUP

Ingredients:
- 300 grams celery, washed and chopped
- 1 small onion, chopped
- 1 1/2 tbsp olive oil
- 2 cups vegetable stock
- 40 grams cashew nuts
- salt and pepper to taste

Instructions:
- Heat the olive oil in a large saucepan then add the celery and onion, stir to coat with oil. Turn the heat low and put the lid on, leaving the vegetables to sweat for 5 minutes.

- Add the garlic, give a quick stir then add the vegetable stock and simmer for 10 minutes.

- Add the cashew nuts to the saucepan and simmer for another 5 minutes or until the celery is cooked through.

- Transfer the soup into a blender and puree until smooth. Season with the salt and pepper and serve.

ANDALUSIAN GAZPACHO

Ingredients:

- 2 pounds very ripe tomatoes, cored and cut into chunks
- 2 pound cucumber, peeled, seeded, and cut chunks
- 1 pound red onion, peeled and cut into chunks
- 1 pound green or red bell pepper, cored, seeded, and cut into chunks
- 4 cloves garlic, peeled and smashed
- 1 teaspoons low sodium salt, plus more to taste
- 1 Cup extra-virgin olive oil, plus more for serving
- 2 tablespoons sherry vinegar, plus more for serving
- 2 tablespoons finely minced chives
- Freshly ground black pepper

Instructions:

- Put all veggies in a large bowl and toss with salt. Let sit till the veggies have released a lot of their liquid.

- Separate the veggies from the liquid, reserving the liquid. Place on a tray and place in the freezer for at least a half hour, or until they are partially frozen.

- Remove from the freezer and let it thaw completely.

- Combine the thawed veggies, reserved juice, oil and sherry vinegar in a large bowl. Ladle into a blender,and blend on high until quite smooth.

- Chill for up to 24 hours. Serve with extra sherry vinegar, olive oil and a sprinkle of chives

MUNCHY MUSHROOM SOUP

Ingredients:

- 1 lb boneless chicken breast, sliced
- 3 cups mushrooms
- 2 large carrots, sliced
- 2 tomatoes, quartered
- 5 cups low sodium chicken stock
- 1 stalk lemongrass, sliced
- juice from 4-6 limes

  2 red chilies, chopped

Instructions:

- Place the chicken stock in a pot, add lemon grass, and bring to boil over medium heat.

- Add the chicken meat, mushrooms, tomatoes, lime juice bring to a boil and simmer for 15 minutes

- Add sugar, chilies, carrots and simmer for an additional 5 minutes. Serve while hot.

TOMATO BASIL SOUP

Ingredients:

- 2 cans whole tomatoes, crushed
- 2 cups tomato juice
- 2 cups low sodium vegetable broth or chicken broth
- 12 or 14 fresh basil leaves
- 1 cup coconut milk
- salt and black pepper to taste

Instructions:

- Combine tomatoes, juice and/or broth in a stockpot. Simmer for 30 minutes.

- Puree, along with basil leaves, in small batches in a food processor, blender or better yet, a hand-held immersion blender right in the pot.

- Return to the pot and add coconut milk while stirring over low heat.

HEALING CHICKEN VEGETABLE SOUP

Ingredients:

- 1 tbsp Coconut Oil
- 1 medium onion, medium dice
- 2 medium carrots, medium dice
- 1 zucchini, medium dice
- 1 medium butternut squash, chopped into cubes
- 12 oz mushrooms, rough dice
- 2-4 cups shredded chicken
- 1 tsp. dried thyme
- 1-2 tsp. dried rosemary + dried basil
- 2-1 tsp. ground cumin
- 1 Tbsp. Apple Cider Vinegar
- salt & pepper to taste
- 6 cups chicken stock

Instructions:

- Heat oil in a large soup pot .Add the vegetables to the pot and stir occasionally.

- Add the chicken ,the herbs, cumin, apple cider vinegar, salt & pepper and stir everything together well.

- Add in your chicken stock .Stir everything up, cover with the lid cracked just a little, and let simmer on low for around an hour .

SAFFRON TURKEY CAULIFLOWER SOUP

Ingredients:
- 1 tbsp extra virgin olive oil
- 1 medium onion, chopped
- 2 large garlic cloves, chopped
- 2 lbs frozen or fresh cauliflower florets
- 1 tsp low sodium salt
- 1 tsp ground black pepper
- 6 cups of water or vegetable broth
- 20 saffron threads
- 1 Diced Turkey Breast

Instructions:
- Saute onion and garlic in olive oil on a soup pot, over medium heat, until onion is translucent, about 10 minutes.

- Add cauliflower florets, low sodium salt and pepper and continue cooking for 10-12 minutes.

- Add 5 cups of water, bring to a boil and simmer until cauliflower is tender, 20-25 minutes.

- Turn off heat. Add saffron, stir and cover. Let the saffron steep for about 20 minutes.

- Blend soup in a blender until creamy. Add Turkey Breast before or after blending

MASALA SOUP

Ingredients:
- 2 tbsp coconut oil
- 1 large onion, chopped
- 4 carrots, chopped
- garlic cloves, chopped
- 1 head of cauliflower, chopped up
- 5 cups low sodium chicken broth
- 1 Diced Turkey Breast
- 1 cup water
- 1 tsp dark mustard seeds
- 1 tsp cumin seeds
- 1 tsp ground coriander
- 1 teaspoon ground turmeric
- 1 tsp low sodium salt
- 1 T lemon juice
- black pepper to taste
- crushed red pepper to taste
- Optional: chopped cilantro on top

Instructions:

- Heat the coconut oil on medium-high and fry the onions, carrots and garlic cloves for about 5 minutes until they are soft.

- Throw in the cauliflower, mustard seeds, cumin, coriander and turmeric. When the cauliflower is soft, add the chicken broth and water and simmer for 10-15 minutes.

- Blend in the food processor until smooth. Simmer for another 10 minutes, add the salt, pepper, lemon juice and crushed red pepper.

- Top with fresh cilantro and add turkey breast

CREAMY CHICKEN SOUP

Ingredients:
- 1/2 cup olive oil
- 2 stalks celery, finely diced
- 2 medium carrots, finely diced
- 5 cups low sodium chicken broth
- 1/2 cup water
- 1 teaspoon dried parsley
- 1/2 teaspoon dried thyme
- 1 bay leaf
- salt to taste
- 3 cups cooked chicken, cubed
- 1 1/2 cups coconut milk or pureed cauliflower

Instructions:
- Place oil in a large soup pot over medium heat. Add the celery and carrots. Cook, stirring occasionally, until soft, 10 to 15 minutes.

- Add broth. If using arrowroot, place it and 1/2 cup cool water in a small bowl or jar and whisk or shake to combine. Add to the pot along with parsley, thyme, bay leaf, and salt.

- Cook, stirring occasionally, until bubbly .Reduce heat, just enough to maintain a boil, and cook, stirring occasionally for 15 minutes.

- Stir in coconut milk (or pureed cauliflower) and chicken and heat through. This is a fairly thick soup; if you like it thinner, add more water, broth, or coconut milk and heat through.

- Remove bay leaf just before serving.

LEMON-GARLIC SOUP

Ingredients:
- 1 tablespoon olive oil
- 1 tablespoon crushed and chopped fresh garlic
- 6 cups low sodium chicken stock
- 2 eggs
- 1/3 to 1/2 cup fresh lemon juice
- 1 tablespoon coconut flour for thickening
- 1/4 teaspoon ground white pepper
- chopped fresh cilantro or parsley, if desired

Instructions:

- In a pot, heat the olive oil over medium-high heat and saute the garlic for 1-2 minutes, or until just fragrant. Do not let the garlic brown.

- Reserve 1/2 cup of the stock to mix with the eggs. Pour the remaining 5 1/2 cups of stock into the pot with the garlic.

- Let the mixture come to a simmer. In a small bowl, whisk together the eggs, lemon juice, arrowroot, white pepper, and half of a cup of reserved stock.

- Pour the mixture into the simmering stock and stir until it all thickens.

- Serve the soup hot, sprinkled with fresh cilantro or parsley.

TURKEY SQUASH SOUP

Ingredients:

- 1 large acorn squash
- 1/2 teaspoon olive oil
- salt and pepper to taste
- 4 cups chicken or vegetable stock
- 1/4 cup coconut milk
- 1-2 turkey breasts shredded
- 3/4 teaspoon ground ginger
- 1 tablespoon coconut aminos

Instructions:

- Preheat the oven to 400. Cut the acorn squash in half and scoop out the seeds and pulp.

- Brush each half with about 1/4 teaspoon olive oil and sprinkle with salt and pepper. Place in a foil-lined baking pan and roast, cut sides up, until fork tender.

- When the squash is cool enough to handle, scoop out the flesh and place it in a medium saucepan, or in a blender if you don't have an immersion blender.

- Add the remaining ingredients and process with an immersion blender or regular blender until smooth.

- Place the saucepan over medium heat and cook, stirring often, until heated through. Serve hot.

ROASTED WINTER VEGETABLE TURKEY SOUP

Ingredients:

- 2 large onions, cut into eighths
- 2 large sweet potatoes, peeled and cut into 1 inch dice
- 1/2 lbs of carrots, peeled and cut into 2 inch dice
- 1 head of garlic, cloves peeled
- 1 tbsp coconut oil
- low sodium salt and pepper to taste
- 2 cups low sodium chicken stock
- 1 turkey breasts

Instructions:

- Preheat the oven to 425 degrees F.

- Distribute the onions, garlic, sweet potatoes and carrots evenly on a sheet tray- it will likely require two trays.

- Top the vegetables with coconut oil. Season GENEROUSLY with low sodium salt and pepper.

- Roast for 25-35 minutes until vegetables are tender, flipping halfway through cooking.

- When the veggies have roasted, transfer them into a large pot on the stove top. Add just enough chicken stock to cover the veggies by 1 inch.

- Put the lid on and bring the liquid to a boil. Reduce the heat and simmer with the lid cracked for 10 minutes.

- Now you get to puree your soup! Taste and season with low sodium salt and pepper if needed.

ZUCCHINI FISH SOUP

Ingredients:

- 4 cups chicken broth
- 3 cups zucchini noodles made with a spiralizer (2 zucchini)
- 2-3 cups cooked sliced white fish of choice
- 2/3 tsp fish sauce
- 1 1/2 tsp grated fresh ginger
- Fresh herbs (handful): basil, mint, cilantro (whichever you prefer)
- Sliced scallions, as much as you like
- Thin slices of jalapeno
- Lime wedges
- Thin slices of red onion

Instructions:

- In a medium-sized pot, heat the broth on medium heat until it becomes steamy.
- Add the ginger, fish sauce and about 2 tablespoons of the herbs.
- Simmer for a few minutes.
- Add your fish, zucchini and cook for about 4 minutes, until your noodles get soft and your meat is warmed.
- Serve with the fresh herbs, jalapeno slices, lime wedges, and red onion slices as you like!

BANANA NUT MUFFINS

Ingredients:
- 2 ripe bananas, mashed with a fork
- 2 eggs
- 1/2 cup almond butter
- 1 tbsp coconut oil, melted
- 1 tsp vanilla
- 1/2 cup coconut flour
- 1 tsp cinnamon
- 1/2 tsp nutmeg
- 1 tsp baking powder
- 1 tsp baking soda
- 1/4 tsp low sodium salt

Instructions:
- Preheat the oven to 350 degrees F. Line a muffin tin with cups. In a large bowl, add bananas, eggs, almond butter, coconut oil, and vanilla. Using a hand blender, blend to combine.

- Add in the coconut flour, cinnamon, nutmeg, baking powder, baking soda, and low sodium salt.

- Blend into the wet mixture, scraping down the sides with a spatula. Distribute the batter evenly into the lined muffin tins, filling each about two-thirds of the way full.

- Bake for 20-25 minutes, until a toothpick comes out clean.

RELISHING RAISIN BREAD

Ingredients:

- 2 room temp eggs
- 1/3 cup melted coconut oil
- 1/3 tsp stevia
- 1/2 cup coconut milk
- 1/2 tsp vanilla extract
- 1/2 cup coconut flour
- 1 tsp cream of tartar
- 1/2 tsp baking soda
- salt (to taste)

For the Swirl

- 1 tbsp water
- 1/2 tbsp cinnamon
- 1 tsp stevia
- A pinch of low sodium salt (to taste)
- 1/4 cup raisins

Instructions:

- Preheat your oven to 325 degrees. Cover the bottom of a loaf pan with parchment paper and grease the sides.

- Separate the eggs - this will allow you to whip up your egg whites and ensure a good light texture.

- Place your egg whites in a medium, clean bowl, and set it aside. Place your egg yolks in a large mixing bowl.

- Add the rest of the wet ingredients to your yolks. Cream until smooth. Add your dry ingredients, mix until well-combined.

- Mix together the first 4 swirl ingredients in a small bowl - Keep your raisins separate.

- With a hand mixer whip up your egg whites until soft peaks begin to form when you remove the beaters. Fold the egg whites into the batter until just combined.

- Add about 1/3 of the batter to your loaf pan - drizzle 1/2 of your swirl, and then quickly with a knife lightly zig-zag the swirl on top of the batter. Sprinkle with half of your raisins

- Add another third of the batter and drizzle the rest of the swirl. Top with the rest of the batter.

- Place in the oven to cook for 47-50 minutes . Remove and let cool for 5-10 minutes. Flip out to complete cooling.

LEMON DELIGHT

Ingredients:
- 2 eggs
- 1/4 cup coconut oil, melted
- 1/3 cup lemon juice
- Zest of 2 lemons
- 1/2 - 1 cup milk (almond or coconut)
- 2/3 cup coconut flour
- 1 heaping teaspoon baking soda
- Pinch of salt

Lemon Glaze
- 1 Tbsp coconut oil
- 1 tbsp water
- 1 tsp stevia
- 1 Tbsp almond milk
- zest and juice from 1 lemon
- 1/2 tsp pure vanilla extract

Instructions:
- Preheat the oven to 350 F.

- Combine all bread ingredients in a mixing bowl and mix well. Pour into a greased pan and bake for 32-45 minutes or until golden on top and the middle is cooked through. Remove from the oven and let cool.

- While the lemon loaf is baking, mix all glaze ingredients together in a small pot over low heat until it starts to simmer.

- Remove from heat and let sit to cool until the lemon loaf is finished cooking and cooling.

- Pour the glaze all over the top of the loaf. Refrigerate the loaf for at least 30 minutes - 1 hour until both the glaze and the loaf firm up a bit.

SWEET POTATO BREAD

Ingredients:
- 2 oz cooked sweet potato flesh
- 1/2 cup coconut flour
- 2 eggs
- 2 tablespoons of coconut milk
- 1 teaspoon baking soda
- Juice of half a lemon
- A pinch of low sodium salt

Instructions:
- Preheat your oven to 350 Degrees Fahrenheit. Grease and line a loaf tin with baking paper hanging over the sides for easy removal.

- Put the ingredients into your food processor or blender and pulse until well combined.

- Spoon the mixture into the prepared tin, smooth over the top with a spoon. Bake for 40 minutes.

- Cover the loaf with foil and bake for a further 20 minutes. Remove from the oven and allow the bread to cool before slicing.

COCONUT LOAF

Ingredients:
- 1/2 cup coconut flour, sifted
- 2 eggs
- zest of one lemon
- 1/2 cup desiccated coconut
- 1 cup coconut yogurt
- 1/2 teaspoon ground cardamom
- 1 cup almond milk
- 1 tsp stevia
- A pinch of low sodium salt
- 1/2 teaspoon concentrated natural vanilla extract
- 1 teaspoon baking soda

Instructions:
- Preheat your oven to 350 degrees Fahrenheit. Grease a mini loaf tin.
- Combine the flour, zest, coconut, baking soda and cardamom. Add the eggs, mix together. Add the yogurt, milk and stevia, combine. Add the salt and vanilla, combine.

- Spoon the mixture into your prepared pan. Bake

for 35 minutes. Cover with foil and bake for another 10 minutes.

- Remove from the oven and allow it to cool slightly before flipping onto a cooling tray.

- Leave to cool for a few minutes before cutting into thick slices.

HEAVENLY HERB FLATBREAD

Ingredients:
- 1/2 cup Coconut Flour
- 2 eggs
- 1 cup coconut milk or almond milk
- 1/2 tsp low sodium salt
- 1/2 tsp dried oregano
- 1/2 tsp dried basil
- 1/2 tsp garlic powder
- drizzle of coconut oil

Instructions:
- Preheat the oven to 375 degrees.

- Mix together the coconut flour, salt, herbs, & garlic powder in a bowl.

- Whisk the eggs and coconut milk in a separate bowl. Pour the wet ingredients into the coconut flour mixture.

- Stir until no lumps are left. Let the batter sit for at least 5 minutes (so the coconut flour absorbs all the liquid). It should resemble a thick paste.

- Prepare your pan. Drizzle some coconut oil on the bottom of the pan and then place the parchment paper.

- Pour out all the mixture into the pan. Cook for 30-40 minutes or until the toothpick comes out clean.

- Allow the bread to cool before transferring it to your container or serving plate.

COCONUT FLOUR MUFFINS

Ingredients:
- 1/2 cup coconut flour
- 2 eggs, at room temperature (that's important)
- 1 cup almond milk
- 2 tsp stevia
- 2 Tbsp. coconut oil
- 2 Tbsp coconut milk at room temperature
- 1 tsp. vanilla extract
- 1/4 tsp. baking soda
- 1 tsp. apple cider vinegar

Instructions:
- Preheat the oven to 350 degrees and prepare a muffin tin with 8 liners.

- Combine the coconut flour and eggs until smooth. Add the remaining ingredients and stir well.

- Divide evenly between the muffin tins. Bake until golden and a toothpick comes out clean, about 20 minutes.

- Cool completely.

CHOCOLATE CAKE

Ingredients:
- 1/2 cup good quality cocoa
- 1/2 cup coconut flour
- 1/2 teaspoons gluten free baking powder
- 1/2 teaspoon ground cinnamon
- Pinch of salt
- 3 eggs
- 1/2 cup coconut oil
- 3/4 cup coconut milk
- 2 teaspoon stevia
- 1 teaspoon vanilla paste

Instructions:
- Preheat the oven to 320°F.

- Combine the cocoa, coconut flour, baking powder, cinnamon and salt into a mixing bowl.

- Add the eggs, stevia, vanilla, coconut milk and coconut oil. Mix well until smooth and combined - a whisk works well for this.

- Pour into a baking tin lined with baking paper.

- Bake the cake for 55 - 60 minutes or until cooked through. Best to test after 45 to make sure as oven temps may vary.

- Remove from the oven and cool. Spread with ganache or healthy chocolate mousse and enjoy.

BLUEBERRY SPONGE ROLL

Ingredients:

- 4 eggs, separated
- 1/3 cup almond milk

- 1/2 cup coconut flour
- 1/2 teaspoon baking soda
- 1/4 teaspoon vanilla powder
- 1 tsp stevia

For filling:

- 1 can coconut cream (chilled in fridge overnight)
- 1 cup blueberry
- A few drops of stevia

Instructions:

- Heat oven to 338 F. Line a Swiss roll pan with baking paper.

- Beat egg whites with electric beaters until they form soft peaks.

- In a separate bowl, beat egg yolks and honey until pale yellow. Add coconut flour, vanilla powder and baking soda to yolks, add milk and stevia and beat until well combined.

- Using a metal spoon, mix 1/3 of the egg white mixture into the egg & flour mixture.

- Gently fold in the remaining egg whites.

- Spread into a lined pan and bake for 12-15 mins until golden brown.

- When the cake comes out of the oven, lift it from the pan using the baking paper.

- Leaving the cake on the paper, start from the short end and roll the cake into a log.

- Place in the fridge to cool with seam side down.

- While the cake is cooling, use electric beaters to beat the coconut cream that has separated to the top of the can and put a few drops of stevia on it. (About 1 cup) After doing the cream, slice blueberries into small pieces.

- After the cake has cooled, unroll and spread the coconut cream and put sliced blueberries at the top of the cake.

LEMON CURD CUPCAKES

Ingredients:
- 1/2 cup coconut flour
- 3 eggs, at room temperature
- 2 tsp stevia
- 1 Tbsp coconut oil
- 2 Tbsp. coconut milk at room temperature
- 1 tsp. vanilla extract
- 1/2 tsp. ground cardamom
- 1/4 tsp. baking soda
- 1/2 tsp. apple cider vinegar
- 3/4 cup stevia sweetened lemon curd

Instructions:

- Preheat the oven to 350 degrees and prepare a muffin tin with 8 liners.

- Combine the coconut flour and eggs until smooth. Add the remaining ingredients and stir well.

- Divide evenly between the muffin tins. Bake until golden and a toothpick comes out clean, about 20 minutes. Cool completely and frost with the lemon curd.

CHOCOLATE RASPBERRY CAKE

Ingredients:

FOR THE CAKE

- 1/2 cup of Coconut Oil
- 1/4 cup of Coconut Flour
- 1/3 cup of Arrowroot Starch
- 1/4 cup of Unsweetened Cocoa Powder
- 1 teaspoon of Baking Soda
- 1/4 cup almond milk
- 1/4 cup of Strong Hot Coffee
- 1 tbsp Stevia
- 2 large Eggs
- 1 teaspoon of Vanilla Extract

FOR THE RASPBERRY SAUCE

- 2 ounces of Raspberries

- 1 teaspoon of Lemon Juice
- 1/4 cup almond milk
- 1 tsp Stevia
- 1/2 teaspoon of Gelatin

FOR THE CHOCOLATE GANACHE

- 2 ounces of Chocolate Chips
- 1/3 cup of Full Fat Coconut Milk

Instructions:

- Whip together the coconut oil and stevia in a large mixer until combined, about 3 minutes on high speed.

- Sift together the coconut flour, arrowroot flour, cocoa powder, and baking soda in a separate bowl. Whisk together the eggs, milk, stevia, coffee, and extract in a large glass.

- Add about a third of the dry ingredients and a third of the liquid ingredients to the mixing bowl and mix until combined. Repeat adding the ingredients in batches until all mixed and uniform.

- Evenly portion the cake batter into muffin tin cups. Bake at 350F for 25-28 minutes, until an inserted toothpick comes out clean.

- Remove from the oven and let the cakes cool for about 10 minutes. Gently remove the cakes from the tin cups using a rubber spatula and set on a cooling rack upside down.

- Gently heat the raspberries, lemon juice, and milk and stevia for about 5 minutes. Remove from heat when the mixture looks uniform. Sprinkle the gelatin on the jam and mix until dissolved.

- Heat the coconut milk to a very low boil. Add to the half of the chocolate chips and mix until fully combined. Then add the rest and mix until uniform.

- Scoop out a portion of cupcake from the center, careful not to puncture it completely. Fill the hole with about a tablespoon of the raspberry sauce. Pour about 2 tablespoons worth directly on top of the raspberry center.

STRAWBERRY DOUGHNUTS

Ingredients:
- 2 large eggs, room temperature
- 2 tablespoons coconut oil, melted
- 1 cup coconut milk, warm
- 1 tsp Stevia
- 1 teaspoon apple cider vinegar
- 1 teaspoon pure vanilla extract
- 1 cup coconut flour
- 1 cup strawberries, grind
- 1 teaspoon baking soda
- 1/2 teaspoon salt

TOPPING

- 1 ounce raw cacao butter, melted
- 2 tablespoons coconut butter
- 1 teaspoon stevia
- 1 cup strawberries, grind

Instructions:

- Preheat a doughnut maker. If using a doughnut pan, preheat the oven to 350 F and grease the pan liberally with butter.

- Using a stand mixer or electric hand mixer, beat the eggs with the coconut oil on medium-high speed until creamy.

- Add the milk, stevia, vinegar, and vanilla and beat again until combined.

- Using a fine mesh sieve or sifter, sift the remaining dry ingredients into the bowl. Beat on high until smooth.
- Scoop the batter into a large Ziploc bag, seal the top, and snip one of the bottom corners.

- Pipe the batter into the doughnut mold, filling it completely. Cook until the doughnut machine indicator light goes off.

- Mix the cacao butter, coconut butter, and stevia in a shallow bowl. Place in the freezer for 5 minutes to thicken.

- Once the donuts are completely cooled, sprinkle ground strawberries on top. Place in the refrigerator for 20 minutes to allow the glaze to set.

PLANTAIN CAKE

Ingredients:
- 2 eggs, separated
- 1 tsp cream of tartar
- 1/2 cup extra virgin coconut oil
- 1/4 cup almond milk
- 1 tsp Stevia
- 1 cup ripe plantain, mashed
- 1 tsp vanilla extract
- 1/2 cup coconut flour, sifted
- 1/2 tsp baking soda
- 1/4 tsp low sodium salt

Instructions:
- Preheat the oven to 350 degrees F. In a bowl combine egg whites and cream of tartar.

- Whip the egg whites until stiff peaks form. In a separate bowl cream together coconut oil, stevia and milk. Do that for a few minutes.

- Add the egg yolks. Mix until smooth. Add mashed plantain and vanilla until mixed.

- Add the sifted coconut flour, baking soda and salt to the egg yolk mixture. Mix until smooth. Slowly add the egg yolk mixture to the whipped egg whites.

- Line a cake tin with parchment paper and grease the sides. Bake for 35 minutes until the top is firm to the touch and a toothpick can be inserted and comes out dry.

LEMON BLUEBERRY CAKE

Ingredients:
- 1 cup coconut flour, sifted
- 3 eggs, beaten
- 1 cup unsweetened coconut milk or almond milk
- 1 tbsp lemon juice
- 1 tbsp lemon zest
- 1 tbsp. coconut oil, melted
- 1 tbsp liquid stevia
- 1 tsp lemon extract .
- 1 tsp baking soda + 1 tsp apple cider vinegar, mixed in scparate bowl
- 1 cup blueberries (optional.)

Lemon Ice Glaze
- 1 tbsp coconut oil, melted
- 1 tbsp coconut butter, melted
- 1 tbsp unsweetened coconut milk
- 2 tbsp lemon juice
- 1 tsp lemon extract
- 1 tsp lemon zest
- 1/3 tsp liquid stevia

Instructions:

- Preheat the oven to 350 F, and grease or oil a round cake pan.

- In a large mixing bowl combine: all the first 8 cake ingredients. Stir together thoroughly; break up any coconut flour lumps. Add in baking soda and vinegar mixture and stir.

- Gently add and mix in the blueberries. Spoon cake batter into the prepared pan and spread around evenly. Bake in a 350 F oven for 30 minutes or until the center is firm. Remove cake from the oven and let cool for 10 minutes while you make the lemon ice glaze.

- Heat a small saucepan over low heat and melt: coconut oil, and coconut butter. Stir the mixture as it melts and break up any coconut butter lumps.

- Once melted, remove from heat and add all the rest of the lemon ice glaze ingredients. Stir the glaze thoroughly until well mixed and set aside to cool.

- Use a large toothpick to poke holes all over the cake. Be sure to poke all the way down to the bottom of the cake.

- Spoon or pour lemon ice glaze all over the top of the cake, making sure to cover well.

- Let the cake cool for a while. It should only take 5 minutes or so for the glaze to solidify a bit. Slice and serve.

COCONUT FLOUR CAKE WITH STRAWBERRY FILLING

Ingredients
- A dozen eggs
- 2 cups coconut milk
- 1 cup milk
- 2 teaspoons Stevia
- 2 teaspoons vanilla extract
- 2 cups coconut flour
- 1/2 teaspoon baking soda
- 1/4 teaspoon salt
- coconut oil for greasing the pan

Strawberry Filling
- 2 cups strawberries, stems removed and sliced

Instructions:
- Place the strawberries in a saucepan over medium heat. After a few minutes, the strawberries will release their juices.

- Allow them to cook uncovered, occasionally

stirring and smashing them. Keep cooking them until the strawberries are soft, smashed and the sauce has reduced.

- Preheat the oven to 350 F. Whisk together the eggs, coconut milk, milk, stevia and vanilla extract. Mix until smooth.

- Add coconut flour, baking soda and salt to the egg mixture and whisk until a smooth batter forms.

- Grease 2 round cake pans with coconut oil.

- Divide up the batter evenly between the 2 cake tins. Use a rubber spatula to smooth it out.

- Bake for 40 minutes, or until a toothpick inserted into the center of the cake comes out clean. Allow the cake to cool.

- Fill the center with the strawberry filling to decorate the cake.

BERRY TRIFLE

Ingredients:
- 1/2 cup plus 2 tsp coconut flour, sifted
- 1/4 tsp low sodium salt
- 1/4 tsp baking soda
- 4 whole eggs (2 of them separated)
- 1/2 cup coconut oil, softened
- 1/2 cup almond milk
- 2 tsp stevia
- 1 tablespoon vanilla extract
- 2 teaspoons lemon juice
- 1 1/2-2 cups diced strawberries
- 1 1/2-2 cups washed blueberries
- 1 1/2-2 cups washed raspberries
- 3-4 cans full-fat coconut milk, cream only

Instructions:

- Preheat the oven to 350 degrees. Sift the dry ingredients together and set aside.

- Separate 2 of the eggs, setting the whites aside and putting the 2 yolks in a medium sized bowl. Crack open the rest of the eggs, adding them to the bowl with egg yolks.

- Using a mixer or hand whisk, beat the coconut oil (liquid or solid, doesn't matter), milk, vanilla and lemon juice until they are well combined.

- On low/medium-speed, mix the dry ingredients into the wet ingredients. Continue to mix till the batter is smooth and has no lumps. Add the eggs (not including the 2 egg whites) in three phases to the batter. Allow each addition to be incorporated completely before adding the next.

- In a small bowl, beat the egg whites till thick soft peaks form. Fold into the batter.

- Pour the batter into a greased square brownie pan or small casserole dish lined with parchment paper, allowing a few inches of flaps to hang over the two long sides of the pan. This will help later with removing the cake to ensure that the sides of the cake won't stick to the pan.

- Bake for 30-45 min. or until a toothpick in the center comes out clean.

- Allow the cake to cool for 5-10 minutes, run a sharp knife along the edges and carefully remove from the pan. Chill 2-3 three cans of full-fat coconut milk (a few hours or overnight).Scoop the thick cream into a medium bowl.

- With a hand/stand mixer, beat the cream on high for a minute or so. Add tsp. stevia as sweetener if desired. Continue beating until well combined.

- Assembly is super easy. Just add some cake to the bottom of your dish, then whipped cream, strawberries/raspberries, whipped cream, more cake, blueberries, more whipped cream, then more fruit if desired or cake crumbles.

LEMON-COCONUT PETIT FOURS

Ingredients:

For the Cake
- 1/2 cup coconut flour
- 1/2 cup coconut milk
- 2 eggs, separated
- 3/4 cup soaked dates in 3 tbsp hot water
- 1/2 tsp vanilla
- 1/2 tsp baking soda
- 1/4 tsp low sodium salt
- 1 tsp lemon rind

Frosting
- 2/3 cup coconut cream (from the top of a can of coconut milk)
- 1 tbsp almond milk
- 1 tbsp Stevia

- 1 tsp lemon juice
- 1/4 cup coconut oil, room temperature

Instructions:

- Put dates in a heat safe bowl or container and pour 3 tbsp boiling water over them and let soak for about 15 minutes.

- Separate the eggs with yolks in one bowl and whites in one large stainless steel, glass or ceramic bowl. When you go to whip the egg whites, it helps if they are at room temperature.

- Once dates have soaked, put them in a food processor along with remaining water and mix until you have a paste-like consistency. Add coconut flour, milk, egg yolks, vanilla, baking soda, salt and lemon rind and mix.Whip the egg whites until foamy and stiff peaks form. This is much easier if you have a stand mixer with the whisk attachment or a hand mixer. It is possible to do it by hand, but it takes time.

- Gently fold egg whites into the batter. Grease a standard sized loaf pan. Put batter in the pan and even out the top with a spatula or spoon.

- Bake in a 350° oven for 20-30 minutes or when a toothpick inserted comes out clean.

- Put coconut cream in a bowl and whisk for a few minutes to make it lighter and creamier.

- Add coconut oil, milk, stevia and lemon juice and

whisk until fully incorporated.

- Allow the cake to cool completely before frosting. Once the cake has cooled, cut small squares or circles out of the cake and skim some cake off of the top with a knife to make it even.

- Cut the squares in half and frost the middle. You can use the prepared frosting, but it will be very thin.

- Drizzle the prepared frosting over the small cake squares and use a spatula or knife to frost the sides evenly. Once you've frosted each petit fours, refrigerate to allow the frosting to harden. Top with a bit of lemon rind.

GINGERBREAD CREAM DELIGHT

Ingredients:

For the Gingerbread Cake
- 1 cup of Coconut Flour
- 1/2 cup of Arrowroot Flour
- 1 teaspoon of Baking Powder
- 1/2 teaspoon of Baking Soda
- 1/2 teaspoon Salt
- 1/2 teaspoon of Ginger Powder
- 1/2 teaspoon of Cinnamon
- 1/2 teaspoon of Nutmeg
- Pinch of Cloves
- 1 cup of almond milk
- 1 teaspoon of Vanilla Extract
- 2 Eggs, room temperature
- 1 cup Coconut Oil
- 1 tsp Stevia

For the Cream Cheese Frosting
- 2 oz Cream Cheese, room temperature
- 1 oz of Coconut oil at room temperature
- 1 tbsp Stevia
- 1 cup of Arrowroot Flour

Instructions:

- Preheat the oven to 350 F and grease a loaf pan.

- Sift together the coconut flour, arrowroot flour, baking powder, baking soda, salt, and spices in a bowl to form the dry mixture.

- Combine the milk and vanilla extract in another bowl to form the liquid mixture.
- Separate the egg whites from the egg yolks.
- Beat the egg whites at high speed in a mixer bowl with a whisk attachment until a meringue forms. Remove the whites from the mixer bowl and set aside.
- Add the coconut oil and coconut sugar to the mixing bowl and beat on medium high for about a minute until uniform.
- Add the egg yolks one at a time to the mixing bowl and beat on medium until combined. Scrape the sides if necessary.
- Add half of the dry mixture to the mixing bowl and beat until combined. Add half of the liquid mixture to the mixing bowl and beat.
- Repeat the previous two steps until all are mixed. Portion a heaping of the egg whites and add to the mixing bowl and mix.
- Fold in the rest of the egg whites until uniform. Pour batter into the loaf pan and bake, centered rack, at 350F for 35 - 40 minutes.
- Whip the coconut oil and cream cheese until smooth. Add the arrowroot flour and stevia. Whip on low until the flour is absorbed into the butter,

then whip on high for a few minutes until light and fluffy.

COCONUT CUSTARD CAKE

Ingredients:
- 3 eggs
- 2 cups almond milk
- 1/2 cup coconut flour
- 1 tsp pure vanilla extract
- 1 tsp baking powder
- 1 tsp stevia
- 1/4 cup coconut, melted
- 1 1/2 cups unsweetened, coconut flakes
- 1/2 cup chocolate chips or broken chocolate bar

Instructions:
- Preheat the oven to 350 F.

- In a large bowl of a stand mixer (or whisk by hand) eggs, milk, coconut flour, stevia, vanilla, coconut oil, and baking powder until smooth. Stir in coconut flakes and chocolate.

- Pour into a cake pan and bake for 45 - 50 minutes. Allow to cool before slicing in the pan. Sprinkle it with cinnamon just before serving.

CRANBERRY ORANGE UPSIDE DOWN

Ingredients:
- 2 cups fresh cranberries
- 1 tablespoon coconut oil (at room temperature)
- 1 teaspoon stevia
- 2 tablespoons coconut flour
- 2 tablespoons arrowroot powder
- 2 teaspoons baking powder
- 1/4 teaspoon salt
- 2 large pastured eggs
- 2 tablespoons melted coconut oil
- 2 tablespoons almond milk
- 2 tablespoons freshly squeezed orange juice
- zest of 1 orange
- 1 teaspoon vanilla

Instructions:
- Preheat the oven to 350 degrees F. Place a sheet of parchment paper onto a cake pan . Grease the sides

of the pan with coconut oil.

- In a small bowl mix together the coconut oil, milk, and arrowroot powder. Spread it onto the cake pan. Arrange the cranberries on top of the mixture.

- In a separate bowl, whisk together the wet ingredients. Pour the wet into the dry and quickly whisk together until combined. Pour batter over fruit and spread evenly with the back of a spoon or spatula.

- Bake for 30 to 35 minutes. Let the pan cool on a wire rack for 15 to 20 minutes then carefully flip out onto a plate; peel off parchment paper. Let cool and then serve. Enjoy!

BAKED VANILLA CARDAMOM DELIGHTS

Ingredients:
- 1/2 cup coconut flour
- 1/8 teaspoon baking soda
- 3/4 teaspoon baking powder
- 1/4 cup Stevia liquid drops
- 1/4-1/2 teaspoon cardamom
- 1 egg, room temperature
- 2 tablespoons coconut oil, liquid (or oil of choice)
- 1/2 cup warm water

Instructions:

- In a bowl place all dry ingredients into a bowl and whisk together. Set aside.

- Next grab your stevia, coconut oil and egg and whisk together in a mixing bowl. Once that is all mixed together add in your dry ingredients. Begin to stir the donut batter.

- End with adding in your warm water to the batter and stir till smooth and combined.

- Preheat your donut maker. Once your green light turns off it is ready. Begin to scoop your donut batter into each donut ring.

- Once all rings are filled close the donut maker and let bake for 2-3 minutes. Repeat process till all our donut batter has been baked.

- Remove donuts from the pan with a knife. Serve and enjoy.

PUMPKIN CREAM COOKIES

Ingredients:

For the donuts
- 5 dried medjool dates, pitted
- 1 cup pumpkin puree
- 1 cup coconut oil, melted
- 2 eggs

- 1 tablespoons coconut flour
- 1 tablespoon cinnamon
- 1 teaspoon nutmeg
- 1/2 teaspoon ground cloves
- 1/2 teaspoon ground ginger
- 1 teaspoon baking powder
- A pinch of salt

For the cream
- 1 (14 ounce) can of coconut cream OR coconut milk refrigerated overnight
- 1 tablespoon stevia
- 1 teaspoon cinnamon

For the chocolate
- 1 cup Chocolate Chips, melted
- 2 tablespoons coconut milk

Instructions:

- Place dried dates in a food processor and pulse to break down.

- Add pumpkin puree, melted coconut oil, and eggs to the food processor and puree until smooth.

- Add coconut flour, cinnamon, nutmeg, ground cloves, ginger, baking powder, and a pinch of salt and puree once more.

- Heat up a donut maker, grease the donut maker or pan, and use the bag to squeeze about 2 tablespoons of the mixture into each donut round.

- In a donut maker, cook for 5-7 minutes. Times will vary with the different donut maker

- Remove donuts once cooked through and let rest and cool on a wire rack.Once cooled, place in the refrigerator for about 10 minutes.

- In a bowl, remove the coconut cream that sits on top of the coconut water and whip together the coconut cream with a fork or whisk. Then add maple syrup and cinnamon and mix well. Place cream in a piping bag or plastic bag and then cut off the end.

- In a bowl, melt chocolate chips and coconut milk that was left behind from the coconut cream via a double boiler or in a microwave.

- Cut the donuts in half, carefully. On the bottom donut, pipe on the cream around the donut then place the top donut half on top of the cream. Then finish the donuts off by dipping them halfway into the melted chocolate.

- Place donuts on a parchment lined baking sheet and into the freezer to harden the chocolate.

SAVORY MUFFINS

Ingredients:
- 1 cup coconut flour
- 1 tsp baking soda

- 2-1 tsp low sodium salt
- 1 cup coconut oil
- 1 cup + 2 tbsp coconut milk
- 2 pastured eggs
- 1 tsp apple cider vinegar
- 1 tsp garlic powder
- 1 tsp each of rosemary, thyme, sage

Instructions:

- Preheat the oven to 350°. Melt the coconut oil and combine with remaining muffin ingredients in a food processor or bowl, mix well.

- Place batter in a muffin tin lined with muffin liners.

- Bake for about 20-30 minutes or until a toothpick inserted comes out clean and the tops are slightly browned. Let it cool and slice in small squares.

LADY FINGERS

Ingredients:

- 2 Pastured Eggs, separated
- 1/4 cup almond milk
- 1/4 tsp Baking Soda
- 1/2 tsp Pure Vanilla Extract
- 1/3 cup Coconut Flour, sifted
- 1 tsp freshly ground Coffee

Instructions:

- Preheat the oven to bake at 400 degrees. Beat egg

whites until stiff in a standing kitchen mixer, or with a hand mixer.

- In a medium sized mixing bowl, combine egg yolks, baking soda, vanilla extract, and milk. Whisk until combined.

- Sift in the coconut flour, and continue to whisk until smooth.Fold in the egg whites, followed by the coffee grounds.

- On a parchment lined baking sheet pipe out 3 inch long cookies with a round piping tube.

- Bake at 400 degrees for 13 minutes, or until cookies are golden brown.

COCONUT CHOCOLATE COOKIES

Ingredients:
- 1/2 cup Virgin Coconut Oil, melted
- 1/4 tsp stevia
- 1/2 tablespoon vanilla extract
- 2 eggs
- 1/8 teaspoon low sodium salt
- 1 cup coconut flour
- 1/2 cup shredded coconut
- 3/4 cup chocolate chips

Instructions:
- Preheat the oven to 375 degrees F.

- Mix together coconut oil, sugar, vanilla, eggs, and salt together. Blend thoroughly. Add flour, coconut and chocolate chips; mix thoroughly.

- Form into small cookies on a parchment lined pan and bake in a preheated oven for about 15 minutes, or until lightly browned.

PEANUT BUTTER PARCELS

Ingredients:
- 1 cup sifted coconut flour
- 1 cup natural peanut butter
- 1 cup peanuts, coarsely chopped (optional)
- 1 tsp Stevia Drops
- 2 eggs
- 1 teaspoon vanilla
- 1/2 teaspoon low sodium salt

Instructions:

- Mix together peanut butter, sugar, eggs, vanilla and salt. Stir in peanuts and coconut flour. Batter will be runny.

- Drop by the spoonful 2 inches apart on a greased cookie sheet. Bake at 375 Degrees F for about 14 minutes.

- Cool slightly and remove from the cookie sheet.

CHOCOLATE PUMPKIN MUFFINS

Ingredients:

- 1 cup pumpkin puree
- 1 cup almond milk
- 1 cup coconut oil, melted
- 2 eggs, whisked
- 1 teaspoon vanilla extract
- 1 cup coconut flour
- 1 teaspoon cinnamon
- 1/2 teaspoon nutmeg
- 1 teaspoon ground cloves
- 1 teaspoon powdered ginger
- 1 teaspoon baking soda
- 1 teaspoon baking powder
- A pinch of low sodium salt
- 1 cup Mini Chocolate Chips
- 1 tsp stevia

Instructions:

- Preheat the oven to 350 degrees.

- Mix together wet ingredients in a bowl: pumpkin puree, milk, coconut oil, eggs, and vanilla extract. In another bowl, whisk together coconut flour, cinnamon, nutmeg, ground cloves, powdered ginger, baking soda, baking powder, and salt.

- Pour dry ingredients into wet ingredients and mix well. Fold in chocolate chips.

- Use an ice cream scoop to scoop batter into 5 silicone baking cups. Bake for 35-40 minutes

SHORTBREAD COOKIES

Ingredients:
- 3/4 cup + 1/2 cup extra coconut flour
- 1/4 cup arrowroot starch
- 1/2 cup coconut oil or butter, melted
- 1/8 tsp low sodium salt
- tablespoons milk
- 1 tsp stevia
- 1/4 cup dark chocolate chips

Instruction

- Preheat the oven to 350 degrees.

- Combine all ingredients except chocolate and 1/2 c extra coconut flour in a mixing bowl. Mush up with a fork and add additional coconut flour until the mixture is crumbly.

- Dust a clean, smooth surface with coconut flour.

Press the crumbly mixture out with your fingers to make it smooth and somewhat flat. Dust with coconut flour.

- Roll the dough to about 1/8-1/4 inch thickness using a rolling pin. Cut shapes out of the dough. Roll the scraps up into a ball and flatten to cut more shapes out.

- Bake on a lightly greased cookie sheet for 15 minutes. Allow the cookies to cool.

- Microwave the chocolate chips for 10 second intervals, stirring between intervals, until they are melted.

- Drizzle cookies with the chocolate. If the chocolate is not very runny, add a tiny amount of coconut oil and stir.

COCONUT PANCAKES

Ingredients:
- 1/4 cup coconut flour
- 1/8 tsp baking soda
- Pinch of low sodium salt
- 1/3 - 1/4 cup coconut milk
- 1 tbsp organic, cold-pressed coconut oil
- 2 eggs
- 1 tsp stevia
- 1/2 tsp vanilla extract
- Coconut oil for cooking

Instructions:

- Thoroughly mix the eggs, coconut oil, and stevia together.

- Add the coconut milk and vanilla extract.Throw in the coconut flour, baking soda, and salt. Mix, but remember, not too much!

- Place a little coconut oil in your skillet and then using a measuring cup, add a little batter to the pan.

- Remember that you aren't likely to see many bubbles forming on the top, so carefully check the underside of your pancake before flipping.

- Serve your pancakes with Blueberry sauce

BLUEBERRY SAUCE

Ingredients:

- 2 cups fresh or frozen blueberries (no need to thaw before use if frozen)
- 1/4 cup water
- 1 tsp. arrowroot powder
- 1 Tbsp water

Instructions:

- Place the berries and 1/4 cup water (or juice) in a small saucepan over medium heat.

- Cook for 5-10 minutes, until bubbling. Slightly

smash some of the blueberries with the back of a fork.

- In a small bowl, stir together the arrowroot powder and 1 Tbsp of water .Remove the saucepan of berries from the heat. While stirring constantly, add the arrowroot mixture into the blueberry mixture.

- Let cool until no longer hot and serve. The sauce will become even thicker when chilled.

FLUFFY COCONUT FLOUR WAFFLES

Ingredients:
- 2 eggs
- 1/2 cup melted butter or ghee (organic and preferably grass-fed)
- 1/2 cup coconut flour
- 1/4 teaspoon low sodium salt
- 1/4 teaspoon baking soda
- 1/4 cup canned coconut milk
- 1 tsp stevia drops

Instructions:
- In a large bowl add the eggs and beat with an electric hand mixer for
30 seconds until the eggs are well beaten.

- Add the melted butter or ghee slowly into the eggs while you are still mixing .Add the coconut flour, pink salt, baking soda and coconut milk.

- Mix with the hand mixer for 45 seconds on low until the batter becomes thicker.

- Heat up your waffle maker and make the waffles according to your maker's specifications.

- Serve with butter, mashed strawberries or maple syrup

FINISH SAVORY PANNUKAKKU

Ingredients:
- 1/4 cup coconut oil
- 1/4 cup coconut flour
- 1/4 cup arrowroot powder
- 1/4 teaspoon low sodium salt
- 1 cup light coconut milk (canned)
- 2 eggs
- 2 teaspoons pure vanilla extract
- 1 tsp stevia

Instructions:
- Preheat the oven to 400 degrees. Place the butter in a 9 by 13 inch baking pan and place it in the oven to let it melt.

- In a medium mixing bowl, stir together the coconut flour, arrowroot, and salt. Whisk in the coconut milk until there are no lumps of starch. Whisk in the eggs, vanilla, and stevia.

- Remove the hot pan from the oven and pour the batter onto the hot butter (pour slowly to avoid splatters of hot butter).

- Return the pan to the hot oven and bake for 15-20 minutes. Serve right away, topped with warmed berries, if desired.

FUDGY COCONUT FLOUR BROWNIES

Ingredients:
- 1/2 cup minus 1 Tbs. coconut
- 1/2 cup cocoa powder
- 1/2 cup plus 2 Tbsp. coconut oil, melted
- 2 eggs, at room temperature
- 1/2 cup almond milk
- 2 Tsp stevia
- tsp. vanilla extract, optional

Instructions:
- Preheat the oven to 300 and grease a glass baking dish (8x8 or 9x9).

- Mix together all ingredients. You can do this by hand or with an electric mixer or high-powered blender.

- Pour into the baking dish and bake for 30-35 minutes, until a toothpick inserted into the center comes out clean. Cool for 30 minutes before cutting or removing from the pan.

PUMPKIN BARS

Ingredients:
- 15 oz. pumpkin puree
- 3/4 cup coconut flour
- 3/4 cup almond milk
- 1/2 teaspoons ground cinnamon
- 3/4 teaspoon ground ginger
- 1/4 teaspoon ground cloves
- 3/4 teaspoon baking soda
- 1/4 teaspoon low sodium salt
- 2 large eggs

Instructions:
- Preheat the oven to 350 F and grease a 9x9" baking dish well with coconut oil.
- Combine all of the ingredients in a large mixing bowl, and stir well until no clumps remain.
- Transfer the batter to the greased baking dish, and use a spatula to smooth the top.
- Bake at 350F for 40-45 minutes, or until the edges are golden and the center is firm.
- Allow to cool completely, then cut into squares and serve.

LEMON BARS

Ingredients:

Crust:
- 2 cups Sifted Coconut Flour
- 1 teaspoon low sodium Salt
- 1 cup almond milk
- 1 tsp stevia
- 16 tablespoons Room Temperature Virgin Coconut Oil {= 1 cup}

Filling:
- 1 cup Fresh Lemon Juice
- 1 cup almond milk
- 1 cup coconut oil
- 1 tsp stevia
- 2 tablespoons Lemon Zest
- 2 Eggs

Instructions:

- Preheat the oven to 350 F. Line a 9x13 inch baking dish with parchment paper.

- Whisk the coconut flour with salt. Thoroughly stir in the milk and coconut oil until it's evenly mixed and crumbly.

- Add the room-temperature coconut oil and stir until it's evenly combined.

- Pat the dough down into the bottom of the baking dish for an even thickness.

- Bake at 350 for approximately 17 minutes or until it starts to brown. Remove from the oven and let cool on the counter while you prepare the filling. Mix stevia with the lemon juice. Working quickly, whisk in the eggs.

- Whisk in the lemon zest. Pour the filling into the now cooled crust.

- Bake at 350 for 25 - 30 minutes or until it's stiffened. Let it cool on the counter for 30 minutes then the refrigerator for 3 hours or overnight.

- Cut into squares and serve chilled.

PUMPKIN BARS

Ingredients
- 1/2 cup coconut manna
- 1/2 cup coconut oil
- 1/4 heaping cup coconut flour
- 1/2 cup cooked winter squash (butternut or pumpkin)
- A pinch of low sodium salt
- 1 tsp. cinnamon
- 1 tsp. ginger
- 1/4 cup almond milk
- 1 tsp stevia

Instructions

- On the stove, gently melt coconut oil and manna until melted.

- In a food processor, add squash, spices, coconut flour, salt, milk and stevia. Pour melted coconut oil and manna on top and blend for 30 seconds being sure all the big pieces of squash are blended.

- Line a square 8x8 brownie pan with parchment paper. Scoop the bar filling into the pan and use a spatula to smooth it out. Bake for 25 min at 350 degrees. Remove from the oven, let cool, cover and put in the fridge until completely chilled; about 3 hours.

COCONUT BISCUITS

Ingredients
- large eggs, yolks and whites divided
- 1/2 cup coconut flour
- 1/4 teaspoon baking soda
- 1/2 teaspoon cream of tartar
- 1/2 teaspoon low sodium salt
- tablespoons coconut oil, room temperature
- 1 tsp stevia

Instructions
- Preheat the oven to 400 degrees.

- In a medium bowl, whisk the egg whites until frothy and at least doubled in size. Mix in the yolks until no streaks remain then add stevia.

- In a separate bowl, combine the flour, baking soda, cream of tartar and salt. Using a fork or pastry cutter, mix the butter into the dry ingredients until you have pea-sized bits of butter.

- Fold the flour mixture into the egg mixture, incorporating well (the batter will be rather wet, but the coconut flour will start to absorb some of the liquid. Do not add more coconut flour!).

- Using a 1/4 cup measuring cup, scoop the batter onto a parchment lined baking sheet.

- Bake for 15-20 minutes or until golden brown and a toothpick inserted into the biscuit comes out clean.

PLANTAIN DROP

Ingredients
- 2 tablespoons coconut oil
- 2 brown plantains (they must be brown)
- 1 tsp stevia
- coconut oil for frying
- 2 eggs
- 1 tablespoon canned coconut milk
- 2 tablespoons coconut flour
- 1-2 teaspoons cinnamon
- 1 teaspoon baking powder
- A pinch of low sodium salt

Instructions

- Preheat the oven to 350 degrees.

- Cut the ends off of the plantains, then use your knife to cut them in half lengthwise and then peel the skin off, cutting off any excess skin that sticks to the plantains. The browner the plantains are, the sweeter they will be and the easier the skin is to take off.

- Now place a large skillet over medium-high heat, add 3 tablespoons of coconut oil to heat up, then add the halved plantains to the skillet. Cook on both sides for about 3-4 minutes until browned, making sure not to burn them.

- Once the plantains are done cooking, add them to the food processor and puree until they begin to clump together.

- Then add the stevia, coconut oil, eggs, and coconut milk and puree until smooth. No clumps should be present at this point.

- Now add coconut flour, cinnamon, baking powder, and salt to the food processor and puree one more time to combine everything well.

- Now line a baking sheet with parchment paper and grab an ice cream scoop to help form perfect sized biscuits.

- Scoop the batter out and plop each biscuit on the baking sheet about 1 inch away from each other.

- Place in the oven and bake for 20-25 minutes until slightly brown and completely cooked through.

ONION HERB COCONUT BISCUITS

Ingredients
- Tbsp. coconut flour
- Tbsp. coconut oil, melted
- 2 eggs
- 1/4 cup very finely minced onion
- 2 garlic cloves, finely minced
- 2 Tbsp coconut milk
- 1 Tbs. fresh chopped herbs (parsley, dill, thyme...) OR 3/4 tsp. dried herbs
- 1/4 tsp. baking soda
- 1/2 tsp. apple cider vinegar

Instructions
- Preheat the oven to 350. Line two baking sheets with parchment paper.

- Mix together the coconut flour, oil, eggs, onion, garlic, yogurt/coconut milk, and herbs. Let sit for 5 minutes; the batter will thicken slightly.

- Mix in the baking soda and vinegar. Drop a spoonful of batter onto the baking sheets. Use the back of a spoon to spread the batter into circles about 1/2" thick. The batter will not spread very much when baking.

- Bake for 12-15 minutes, until moist but cooked through. Cool at least 10 minutes before serving, or they will be too crumbly.

ONION BISCUITS

Ingredients
- 1/3 cup coconut flour
- 1 cup coconut oil, melted
- 2 eggs
- 1/4 tsp low sodium salt
- 1/4 tsp cream of tartar
- 1/8 tsp baking soda
- 1 cup shredded onion

Instruction
- Preheat the oven to 400 degrees. Put flour, salt, cream of tartar and baking soda in a small bowl

- Put eggs and coconut oil in a mixing bowl, and whisk until smooth

- Add flour mixture, and whisk until no lumps remain. Stir in the onion.

- Drop by spoonful onto a lightly oiled baking sheet. Bake for 8-10 minutes until lightly browned.

CRISP COCONUT FLOUR TORTILLAS

Ingredients

- 1/2 cup coconut flour
- 1/2 teaspoon grain free baking powder
- 1/4 teaspoon low sodium salt
- 1/2 cup egg whites
- 3/4 cup almond milk

Instruction

- Mix all of the ingredients in a bowl.

- Let it sit for 10 minutes so the coconut flour can soak up some of the moisture, and then whisk again. The batter should be runnier than that of pancakes, about the same as a crepe batter.

- Heat a non-stick skillet over medium high heat and spray with oil or melt enough butter to coat the bottom and sides of the pan.

- Pour 1/4 cup of the batter into the pan, swirling the pan while you pour to ensure the bottom is coated and the tortilla is thin.

- Once the bottom looks set (about 1 minute), carefully release the sides of the tortilla with a rubber spatula and turn over.

- Spray the pan again, and repeat the above steps until all the batter is used. Layer the tortillas on a plate and set aside until you're read to fill them and bake.

EASY PIZZA CRUST RECIPE

Ingredients

- 1 cup tapioca flour (starch) (plus more for rolling out dough)
- 1/3 cup + 2-3 tablespoons coconut flour, separated
- 1 teaspoon low sodium salt
- 1/2 cup olive oil
- 1/2 cup warm water
- 1 large egg, whisked

Instructions

- Preheat oven to 450 degrees F

- Combine the tapioca flour (you can substitute arrowroot flour/starch), salt and 1/3 cup coconut flour in a medium bowl.

- Pour in oil and warm water and stir. Add the whisked egg and continue mixing until well combined.

- Add two to three more tablespoons of coconut flour - one tablespoon at a time - until the mixture is soft but somewhat sticky dough.

- Turn out the dough onto a surface sprinkled with tapioca flour and knead it gently until it is in a manageable ball that does not stick to your hands.

- Place the pizza dough ball onto a sheet of parchment paper. Use a tapioca floured rolling pin to carefully roll out the dough until it is fairly thin. You may end up using another few tablespoons of tapioca at this point. You will need it to keep the dough from being too sticky. But don't overwork the dough or add TOO much more tapioca or your dough will be too dense.

- Place the rolled out dough (on its parchment paper) into the preheated oven onto a hot pizza stone or sheet pan. Bake for 12-15 minutes.

COCONUT PIZZA CRUST

Ingredients
- 1 egg
- 1 tablespoon cream of buckwheat
- 1 tablespoon coconut flour
- 1/8 teaspoon baking soda

Instructions
- Preheat the oven to 425. Mix all ingredients in a bowl until well combined.

- Line a cookie tray with parchment paper and spread the cheese mixture on the paper as thinly as possible, using the back of a spoon or fork.

- Reduce heat to 400 and bake on the top rack for about 15 minutes, or until the crust is starting to look golden in places. Remove from the oven and add desired toppings.

CREAMY CROISSANT

Ingredients
- 2 eggs, separated.
- 1 tsp cream of tartar, where to buy this
- 1 tbsp organic coconut cream, softened.
- 2 tbsp coconut oil, melted
- 2 tbsp coconut flour
- 15 drops liquid stevia

- tsp baking soda + 1 tsp cream of tartar, mix together in a separate pinch bowl.
- 1 tsp low sodium salt

Instructions

- Preheat the oven to 300 F, and grease or oil a bagel or donut pan.

- Separate egg whites from yolks, and place whites in one mixing bowl, and yolks in another mixing bowl.

- Add cream of tartar to egg whites and whip with a stand mixer or hand mixer until stiff peaks form. Set aside.

- Beat egg yolks in a separate mixing bowl and add: creamed coconut, melted coconut oil, coconut flour, stevia, baking soda and cream of tartar mixture, and sea salt. Beat egg yolk mixture until thoroughly combined.

- Gently fold egg yolk mixture into egg white mixture until combined (careful not to stir or beat (should still be a whipped meringue texture).

- Spoon mixture into bagel pan, and spread around, with the back of a spoon, in the pan.

- Bake for 20 to 25 minutes or until the tops and edges are slightly browning. Should check at 20 minutes, as all oven temperatures can vary.

GNOCCHI BALLS

Ingredients

- 2 eggs, beaten
- 1 tbsp coconut flour
- 1 tsp garlic powder
- 1/4 tsp low sodium salt

Instructions

- Mix the coconut flour and beaten eggs well. Add the garlic powder and salt and mix well into the dough.

- Place the dough on a sheet of cling film and roll into a long sausage shape.

- Wrap up with the cling film and place in the refrigerator. Chill the dough for a minimum of 30 minutes.

- Bring a saucepan of water to the boil.

- Remove the Gnocchi dough from the refrigerator and cut into small bite sized pieces.

- Place the pieces into the boiling water, reduce the heat to medium and cook for 4-5 minutes. Remove with a slotted spoon. Repeat until all gnocchi are cooked.

- Top with the sauce of your choice.

CRISPY COCONUT CRACKERS

Ingredients

- 4 ounces shredded coconut
- 2 oz tablespoons butter, softened
- 1/4 cup tapioca flour
- 1 tablespoon coconut flour
- 1/2 teaspoon baking soda
- 1/4 teaspoon powdered mustard
- 1/4 teaspoon powdered onion

Instructions:

- Preheat your oven to 350 F. Line a baking sheet with parchment paper or a silicone mat.

- Combine all ingredients in a food processor. Buzz until a ball of dough has formed.

- Use your hands to shape dough into 1-inch balls. Place balls on the baking sheet, leaving about 3 inches of space between each.

- Bake until the edges are slightly browned, about 10 minutes.

CUSTARD PIE

Ingredients
- 3 Eggs
- 2 cups coconut milk
- 1/4 cup coconut oil (softened works best)
- 1/2 cup almond milk
- 2 tsp stevia
- 1/2 cup coconut flour
- 1/2 teaspoon baking powder
- 1/2 teaspoon low sodium salt
- 1 tablespoon vanilla (or 2 vanilla beans scraped)
- 1 cup shredded dried coconut

Instructions
- Preheat the oven to 325 degrees F.

- Place all ingredients into a blender and blend for about 10 seconds.

- Pour into a pie dish greased with coconut oil.

- Bake for 55 minutes in a preheated oven. Serve warm (or cold the next day for breakfast!)

PALEO TORTILLAS

Ingredients

- 1/4 cup coconut flour
- 1/4 teaspoon baking powder
- 1 cup egg whites
- 1/2 cup water
- A pinch of low sodium salt
- coconut oil (as needed, for greasing the press or pan)

Instructions

- In a bowl mix all ingredients. Set aside for five minutes. The batter takes about that long to hydrate and thicken.

- In a preheated electric tortilla press: Pour about a little less than 1/4 cup of batter onto the tortilla press. Quickly smooth out using a heat resistant spoon, and press the top of the press down to distribute the rest of the batter. Cook until the indicator on the press goes off.

- In a pan over medium heat: Pour a little less than 1/4 cup of batter onto the pan. Quickly smooth out using a heat resistant spoon.

- Cook for 1 to 2 minutes or until the edges of the tortilla start to turn golden brown. Then flip and cook for an additional minute or two.

- Transfer tortillas to a plate and cover with a paper towel to keep warm.

- Serve with desired toppings

CHOCOLATE-CARAMEL BROWNIES

Ingredients

- 1/4 cup coconut flour
- 1 1/4 cup cacao powder
- 2 eggs
- 1 teaspoon low sodium salt
- 1 teaspoon baking soda
- 1/2 cup almond milk
- 1 tsp stevia
- 1 tablespoon vanilla extract
- 1/3 cup coconut oil
- 1/3 cup dark chocolate chips
- Keto friendly caramel sauce

Instructions:

- Preheat the oven to 350 degrees Fahrenheit.

- Mix dry ingredients in one bowl and wet ingredients in a second bowl.

- Combine both mixtures and stir until all ingredients are incorporated together.

- Pour the mixture into a greased 8x8 pan.

- Top with chocolate chips and/or nuts if desired, and bake for 25-30 minutes.

- Let cool and then drizzle with caramel sauce.

CINNAMON APPLE MUFFINS

Ingredients:
- 1 cup unsweetened applesauce
- 2 eggs
- 1/4 cup coconut oil, melted
- 1 tsp vanilla
- Stevia to taste
- 1/2 cup coconut flour
- 1 tsp cinnamon
- 1/2 tsp baking powder
- 1/2 tsp baking soda
- 1/4 tsp low sodium salt

Instructions:
- Preheat the oven to 350 degrees F. Line a muffin tin with liners. In a large bowl, add applesauce, eggs, coconut oil, stevia, and vanilla. Stir to combine.

- Stir in the coconut flour, cinnamon, baking powder, baking soda, and low sodium salt. Distribute the batter evenly into the lined muffin tins, filling each about two-thirds of the way full.

- Bake for 15-20 minutes, until a toothpick

inserted into the center comes out clean. Serve warm or store in the refrigerator in a resealable bag.

CHOCOLATE HAZELNUT CUPCAKES

Ingredients:

- 1 large (or 3 medium) zucchini, grated (about 3 cups grated)
- 2 eggs
- 2 cups Hazelnuts
- 6 drops stevia liquid (May need a few more - please taste test)
- 1/4 cup coconut oil (room temperature)
- 1/3 cup Tapioca Flour (this is the same thing as Tapioca Starch)
- 1/4 cup cocoa powder
- Tsp Vanilla Extract
- 1 tsp Baking Soda
- 1 tsp Salt

Instructions

- Preheat the oven to 350 F. Line a muffin pan with paper liners, use Silicone Muffin Cups. or bake in a silicone muffin pan.

- Grind hazelnuts in a Food Processor or Magic Bullet until they are super fine and almost turning into hazelnut butter.

- Finely grate zucchini (you could even process in a food processor).

- Combine ground hazelnuts, grated zucchini and the rest of the ingredients together in a bowl. The batter is quite runny. That's okay- that's why these cupcakes are so fudgy.

- As an alternative you can combine all ingredients in a food processor or blender and process/blend until smooth.

- Pour mixture into prepared muffin pan and bake for 30 minutes. Let cool completely before icing or serving. Enjoy!

BURSTING BANANA CUPCAKES WITH SESAME FROSTING **Ingredients**

FROSTING
- 1 oz cocoa butter
- 1 vanilla bean
- 4 drops stevia liquid
- 1/4 cup tahini (sesame seed butter)
- 1 tsp arrowroot powder
- 1/4 cup room temperature coconut oil

CUPCAKES
- 2 large (or 4 medium) overripe bananas
- 2 eggs
- 1 Tbsp extra virgin coconut oil

- 4 drops stevia liquid (May need a few more - please taste test)
- 1 tsp vanilla
- 1/3 cup coconut flour
- 1/3 cup arrowroot powder
- 1 tsp baking soda
- 1/8 tsp low sodium salt

Instructions

- Cut the vanilla bean lengthwise and scrape out the vanilla seeds with a sharp knife (save the pod for making vanilla ice cream or some other dish where you simmer the vanilla pod in coconut milk).

- Add cocoa butter. Add stevia to melted cocoa butter and whisk until cane juice has dissolved. Add the remaining ingredients and whisk together until fully combined.

- Allow to cool to room temperature (because of the high melting point of cocoa butter, this takes a long long time-if you want to speed it up, put it in the fridge and whisk aggressively every 5 minutes while it cools). Whisk every so often just to make sure it doesn't separate or clump up.

- Preheat the oven to 350 F.

- Grease a muffin pan or put paper liners. I actually use a silicone muffin pan just because it's so easy and ends up saving me tons of time!

- Combine all of the ingredients in a blender or food processor (yes, it really is that easy). Blend or process about 1-2 minutes until you have a thick and smooth batter.

Pour batter into the prepared muffin pan. You can make your cupcakes a bit bigger by dividing into 10 muffin cups or a bit smaller by dividing into 12 muffin cups.

- Bake for 40 minutes (45 if you only make 10). Remove from the oven and let cool completely before frosting. Enjoy!

LEMON CUPCAKES WITH LEMON FROSTING

Ingredients

Lemon Coconut Butter Frosting
- 1 cup fresh Lemon Juice
- 1 cup coconut cream butter
- 5 drops stevia liquid

Cupcakes
- 1 cup Coconut Flour
- 1 cup Tapioca Flour
- 1 tsp Baking Soda
- 2 Eggs
- 6 drops stevia liquid (May need a few more - please taste test)
- 1 cup fresh Lemon Juice (roughly juice of two lemons)
- 1 Tbsp finely grated Lemon Zest (roughly zest from two lemons)

Instructions

- Preheat the oven to 350 F. Line a muffin tin with paper muffin cup liners. Blend all ingredients together until a smooth batter forms.

- Let the batter rest for 2-3 minutes to thicken. Pour batter into the prepared muffin tin.

- Bake for 22-23 minutes, until starting to turn golden brown along the edges.

- Carefully remove cupcakes from the pan and cool on a wire rack. Let cupcakes cool completely before frosting.

- Mix coconut cream concentrate, lemon juice and stevia until thoroughly combined. Spread a generous amount of frosting (whichever you choose) on each cupcake. Candied lemon zest and edible flowers make great decorations for these cupcakes.

RED VELVET CHOCOLATE CUPCAKES WITH COCONUT- CHERRY GLAZE

Ingredients

- 1 cup beets, peeled and finely grated
- 1 1/2 cup blanched almond flour
- 1 teaspoon baking soda
- 2 tablespoons raw cacao powder
- 1 cup coconut oil, melted

- 3 tablespoons coconut milk, full fat
- 1 teaspoon vanilla extract
- 1 teaspoon apple cider vinegar
- 2 tablespoons raw stevia
- 1 egg
- 1 cup chocolate chips

COCONUT-CHERRY GLAZE

- 1 can coconut milk, full fat
- 1 teaspoon vanilla extract
- fresh cherries, pitted

Instructions

- Preheat the oven to 350°F and line a muffin tin with baking cups. Mix together the blanched almond flour, baking soda and raw cacao powder.
- In a separate bowl, whisk together the coconut oil, coconut milk, vanilla extract, apple cider vinegar, stevia, egg and grated beets.
- Using a rubber spatula, gently mix the wet and dry ingredients together. Fold chocolate chips into the batter.
- Spoon batter into prepared muffin tin, filling each to the top.
- Bake until a toothpick inserted into the center comes out clean, about 30- 35 minutes.
- Set the pan on a wire rack to cool, then top with

the coconut glaze and a fresh cherry.

- Place a can of full fat coconut milk in the fridge overnight. Scoop the coconut cream that forms on top of the can into a bowl, being careful not to mix with the water in the bottom of the can.

- Add the vanilla extract and using a handheld or stand electric mixer, whip the coconut cream until fluffy.

- Garnish your cupcakes and enjoy!

PINK VELVET CUPCAKES WITH VANILLA FROSTING

Ingredients

Cupcakes
- 1/2 cup coconut oil
- 4 drops stevia liquid
- 2 eggs
- 1 teaspoon vanilla extract
- 3/4 cup almond flour
- 1/2 cup coconut flour
- 1 teaspoon baking powder
- 2 tablespoons beet powder (optional)

Frosting
- 1/2 cup room temperature coconut oil
- 5 drops stevia liquid
- 1 teaspoon vanilla extract
- 2 tablespoons almond

- 2 teaspoons coconut flour
- 1 tablespoon chilled canned coconut milk fat

Instructions:

- Preheat the oven to 350 degrees Fahrenheit.In a stand mixer or large bowl, mix together coconut oil, stevia, eggs and vanilla extract with a mixer or whisk.

- In a separate bowl, whisk tapioca flour, coconut flour, baking powder, beet powder and salt together

- Slowly mix the dry mixture in with the wet mixture, adding 1 cup at a time until well mixed

- Scoop your batter into muffin liners in a muffin pan. Fill each well 2/3 of the way and you should get 10 cupcakes.Place in the oven and bake for 18-20 minutes or until cooked through. Use a toothpick to poke through a muffin to make sure the toothpick comes out clean.

- Combine the coconut oil shortening, stevia, vanilla, almond flour and coconut flour in the bowl of a stand mixer with a whisk attachment or a large mixing bowl.

- Using the stand mixer or a hand mixer, beat until smooth.

- Add your chilled coconut milk and beat until well combined. Do not over mix or your frosting might separate . Once your cupcakes are completely cool, use immediately by placing in a piping bag or Ziploc bag with a corner cut off to frost your cupcakes

PALEO BANANACADO FUDGE CUPCAKES

Ingredients

- 1/2 cup almond butter
- 1/4 cup stevia
- 1 ripe bananas
- 2 medium avocados
- 2 eggs, beaten
- 3/4 cup cocoa powder
- 1 tbsp. vanilla
- 1 tsp baking soda
- 1 tsp baking powder

Instructions

- In a large bowl, mix the almond butter and stevia.

- In a blender or mixer, beat the eggs, banana, vanilla, cocoa powder and avocado to form a mousse-like consistency.

- Add baking soda and baking powder. Fold into the almond butter to make batter.

- Pour into a mini-cupcake tin . Bake at 350 for 15-18 minutes depending on size and desired consistency.

CHOCOLATE CUPCAKES WITH COCONUT CREAM FILLING

Ingredients:

Cupcakes
- 1/4 cup coconut flour
- 1/4 cup organic cocoa powder
- 2 large eggs
- 1/4 cup coconut oil
- 6 drops stevia liquid
- 1/4 tsp baking soda
- 1 tsp lemon juice
- Pinch of salt

Filling (Optional)
- 13.5 oz can of full fat coconut milk
- 4 drops stevia liquid (May need a few more - please taste test)
- 1 tsp vanilla extract

Chocolate Frosting
- 2 ripe avocados
- 1/2 cup organic cocoa powder
- 5 drops stevia liquid (May need a few more - please taste test)
- 1 Tbsp coconut oil, melted

Instructions:

- Preheat the oven to 350 F. Combine the coconut flour, cocoa powder, sweetener, baking soda, and low sodium salt.

- In a separate bowl, combine the eggs, coconut oil, and lemon juice.

- Add the dry ingredients to the wet and mix to combine. Line a muffin tin with 7 cupcake liners.

- Fill cupcake liners evenly with the batter and bake for 18 - 20 minutes or until cooked through.

- Combine the coconut cream, sweetener, and vanilla and mix until smooth. Pipe the cream into the hole cut out of the cupcake.

- Place the meat of the avocados in a mixer and mix until completely smooth.

- Add the cocoa powder and sweetener and mix until thoroughly incorporated. Add the butter and mix to combine.

- Allow to cool before filling with cream and topping with the icing. Once cool, cut a small hole in the middle of each cupcake, reserving the lid/top of the hole that was cut out.

- Fill with cream and place the lid/top back on the cupcake to cover the hole. Pipe chocolate frosting (directions below) onto each cupcake and serve.

APPLE PIE CUPCAKES WITH CINNAMON FROSTING

Ingredients:

- 2 Eggs, room temperature
- 1/2 cup applesauce
- 5 drops stevia liquid (May need a few more - please taste test)
- 1/3 cup coconut oil, melted
- 1/4 cup finely ground blanched almond flour
- 1/2 cup coconut flour
- 1/2 tsp. low sodium salt
- 1/2 tsp. baking powder

Frosting

- 1 cup coconut oil
- 4 drops stevia liquid
- 1 tsp. cinnamon
- Dash of salt

Instructions:

- Preheat the oven to 350 F. Line muffin pan with baking cups. Combine all wet ingredients in a medium sized mixing bowl. Beat on medium with a hand mixer for about 30 seconds.

- Combine all dry ingredients in another medium sized bowl. Mix together with a fork to break apart any clumps. Add the dry ingredients to the wet ingredients and beat for about 20 seconds. Make sure all ingredients are combined.

- Fill each lined muffin tin about 3/4 of the way full. Bake for 25-30 minutes or until a toothpick comes out clean in the center.

- Combine all of the ingredients into a medium mixing bowl and beat on medium speed for about 30 seconds until well combined. Ice those cupcakes and get to eating!

PALEO STICKY DATE PUDDING CUPCAKES

Ingredients

For the muffins
- Coconut Butter grease the muffin tray with
- 3 tbsp water
- 5 dates
- 1 ripe banana, peeled and roughly chopped
- 3 tbsp coconut flour
- 1 tbsp vanilla extract
- 2 eggs
- 5 drops stevia liquid
- 1 tsp baking powder

For the sticky date ganache
- 5-6 dates, chopped
- 1 tbsp of orange juice
- 1 tbsp almond milk (coconut milk or water can also be used)
- 1 tsp vanilla extract or essence
- 4 drops stevia
- Fresh raspberries or strawberries for garnish

Instructions

- Preheat the oven to 365 °F. Grease muffin tins with the butter and set aside.

- Heat the dates and water in a small saucepan over low heat until the dates break down and thicken. Use a fork to mash them together and set aside.

- Place the coconut flour, egg, banana, vanilla extract and baking powder in a blender or food processor and mix well until well combined and aerated.

- Add the dates to the banana mixture and combine. Evenly distribute into the ramekins. Cook in the oven for about 20-22 minutes.

- While the muffins are in the oven, place the sticky date ganache ingredients in a small saucepan over a low heat and cook for about 3-4 minutes or until the dates break down. Mash with a fork and whisk until thickened. Set aside.

- Allow the muffins to rest for 5 minutes before removing them to a serving plate. Scoop a dollop of sticky date ganache paste on top and garnish with a few raspberries.

PUMPKIN COCO CUPCAKES WITH CREAMY CINNAMON FILLING

Ingredients

- 1 cup pumpkin puree
- 2 eggs
- 5 drops stevia liquid (May need a few more - please taste test)
- 1 Tbsp raw apple cider vinegar
- 1 Tbsp melted butter or coconut oil
- 1 tsp vanilla extract
- 2 cups almond flour
- 1 Tbsp coconut flour
- 1 tsp cinnamon
- 1 tsp cardamom powder
- 1/2 tsp ginger powder
- 1 tsp each nutmeg, allspice and cloves
- 1/4 tsp sea low sodium salt
- 1 tsp baking soda
- 1 oz unsweetened baking chocolate (can also use chocolate chips)

Frosting:

- 1 cup Full fat creamed coconut
- 1 cup coconut butter, softened
- 5 drops stevia liquid (May need a few more - please taste test)
- 1 tsp vanilla extract
- 1 Tbsp cinnamon

Instructions

- Preheat the oven to 350 F. Line a cupcake pan with liners.

- In a medium bowl, whisk together the pumpkin puree, eggs, stevia, butter and vanilla extract. Mix until smooth. Add in the flours, spices, low sodium salt and baking soda and stir until well combined. Add the vinegar. Using a sharp knife, cut the baking chocolate into small chunks. Fold into the cupcake batter to evenly distribute.

- Portion out into lined cupcake tins, until they are almost completely full of batter; these will not rise very much, so no need to worry too much about them getting too big.

- Bake for 25 minutes. Check with a toothpick to make sure they are done; if the toothpick comes out clean, they are ready. If not, add 5 more minutes to the baking time. Let cool completely before frosting.

- Using a strong fork, cream together the cream and butter until smooth. Stir in the stevia, vanilla and cinnamon, and stir well until creamy and well combined.

- Use a piping bag or simply a knife to top the cooled cupcakes with the buttercream frosting.

BANANA CHOCO CUPCAKES

Ingredients:
- 2 cups almond meal
- 1/2 cup almond butter
- 2 ripe bananas
- 1/4 cup cocoa powder, unsweetened of course
- 1/2 cup coconut sugar
- 1/2 cup chocolate chips
- 2 eggs
- 1 tsp pure organic vanilla extract
- 1 tsp low sodium salt
- 1/2 tsp baking soda
- 1 tsp apple cider vinegar

Instructions

- Instead of mixing wet and dry ingredients separate from each other, just build it all in one bowl.

- Preheat the oven to 350 degrees. Mash the bananas, mix in the almond butter and coconut palm sugar, add the vanilla extract, salt, eggs, baking soda and vinegar. Make it chocolaty and dump in the cocoa powder. Mix that in well and start adding the almond meal a cup at a time to make sure it all incorporates well.

- Line a muffin pan with the paper liners, fill each cup with batter. Bake for 20 minutes and let cool before eating.

JAM & CREAM

CUPCAKES *Cupcakes*

- 1/2 cup coconut flour, sifted
- 1/4 cup almond flour
- 2 eggs
- 5 drops stevia liquid
- 2 tablespoons coconut oil
- 1 cup full fat coconut cream
- 1/2 teaspoon concentrated natural vanilla extract
- 1 teaspoon baking powder

Sugar free strawberry jam

- 1 heaped cup of chopped strawberries
- 2 tablespoons chia seeds
- 2 drops stevia

   Cream

- cup raw macadamia
- 1/2 teaspoon vanilla extract

Instructions

- Place the cream ingredients into your blender or

food processor and blend at high speed until you have a lovely, smooth macadamia butter.

- Place the jam ingredients into a blender or food processor and blend until smooth and well combined. Pour / spoon the mixture into a container and place in the fridge to thicken.

- Preheat your oven to 175 degrees Celsius or 350 degrees Fahrenheit

- Line nine holes of a standard muffin tray with cupcake cases.

- In a medium sized bowl, beat together your stevia and coconut oil.

- Add in the eggs, coconut cream and vanilla. 5. Add the flours and when smooth and well combined gently add the salt and baking powder.

- Spoon the mixture evenly into your nine cases. Bake for 25 minutes.

- Allow to cool slightly before moving from the tray to a cooling rack.

- Leave the cakes to cool completely before using a small, sharp knife to remove the tops of the cupcakes and create a small indent in the cake.

- Fill the cake with a teaspoon of jam and a

teaspoon of 'cream'. Gently place the cupcake 'lid' back on top.

YELLOW CUPCAKE

RECIPE **Ingredients**

- 1 cup of sifted coconut flour
- 2 large eggs
- 1 cup of butter or ghee or coconut oil
- 1 teaspoon vanilla
- drops stevia liquid
- 1 cup of applesauce
- 1 teaspoon baking powder
- 1 teaspoon baking soda

Instructions:

- Combine the coconut flour, baking powder and baking soda in a bowl and blend.

- Add in all the liquid ingredients; mix well with a spoon.

- Pour into the cupcake tins and bake at 350 degrees for 20 minutes.

- Frost and enjoy!

PEAR & NUTMEG CUPCAKES

Ingredients

- 3 ripe pears, peeled, de-cored and chopped into small pieces
- 1/2 tsp nutmeg
- 2 tbsp water
- 1/4 cup coconut flour
- 2 large eggs
- 1/4 cup coconut oil or melted butter
- 5 drops stevia liquid
- 1/4 tsp baking powder

Instructions

- Add the pear, water, 5 drops of stevia and 1/2 tsp of nutmeg to a saucepan. Let the mixture simmer over a medium heat until the pears soften (about 15 mins). Either mash with a hand-masher or transfer to a blender and puree. Set aside to cool.

- Sieve the coconut flour, the remaining tsp of nutmeg and baking powder into a mixing bowl. In a separate bowl, beat the eggs, coconut oil/butter and stevia together.

- If the pear puree is cool, stir it into the eggs.

- Gradually add the wet ingredients to the dry and stir until it forms a semi- runny batter.

- Spoon into a muffin tray (it should make 6 muffins). Bake at 375 for 12-15 mins.

VANILLA PALEO CUPCAKES

Ingredients:
- 2 tbsp Coconut Oil
- 1 cup Unsweetened Applesauce
- 2 Eggs
- 1 teaspoon Vanilla Extract
- 4 drops stevia liquid
- 1 cup Almond Flour
- 2 teaspoons Cinnamon
- 1 teaspoon Baking Powder
- 1/8 teaspoon low sodium Salt

Cinnamon Frosting:
- 1 cup room temperature coconut oil
- 5 drops stevia liquid
- 2 tablespoons almond flour
- 2 teaspoons Coconut Flour
- 2 teaspoons Cinnamon
- 2 tablespoons Chilled Coconut Milk Cream
- 1 Apple Thinly Sliced
- Cinnamon for Dusting

Instructions
- Preheat the oven to 350 degrees F. Line a mini cupcake pan with 24 paper liners.
- Melt the butter then whisk in with the applesauce, eggs, vanilla, and stevia.

- Add the almond flour, cinnamon, baking powder, and salt to the wet ingredients and mix until evenly combined.Evenly distribute into the 24 mini cupcake liners {about 1 tablespoon of batter each} and bake at 350 F for 18 - 19 minutes.

- Let cool completely.

- Whisk the shortening, stevia, vanilla, arrowroot, coconut flour, and cinnamon together until smooth.

- Add the chilled coconut milk cream and whisk again until smooth.

- Use immediately. Either spoon the frosting into a gallon plastic bag or a pastry bag.

- Gently frost each cupcake with your desired amount of frosting.

- Store the rest of the frosting in the refrigerator. Let it come to room temperature before you use it as frosting again.

- Top each cupcake with a thin slice of fresh green apple and dust with ground cinnamon

CHOCOLATE CHIP CUPCAKES

Ingredients

- 1/2 cup Coconut Flour
- 2 Eggs
- 2 Egg Whites
- 1/2 cup Cashew Butter (or coconut oil for nut free)
- 1/2 tsp low sodium Salt
- 1/2 tsp Baking Soda
- 1/2 tsp Baking Powder
- 6 drops stevia liquid
- 3/4 cup Egg Nog
- 1/4 tsp Vanilla
- 1/2 t Nutmeg
- 1 cup Chocolate Chips
- Vanilla frosting for garnish

Instructions

- Whisk together the dry ingredients.
- Beat the eggs, whites, eggnog, butter, vanilla, and stevia.
- Add the dry mixture and whisk until smooth. Fold in the chocolate chips.
- Preheat the oven to 350 degrees. Fill lined muffin tins 1/2 full with batter. Bake for 25-30 minutes, or until a toothpick.

BOSTON CREAM PIE CUPCAKE

BONANZA *VANILLA CREAM*

Ingredients:

- 2 egg yolks
- 5 drops stevia liquid
- 4 tablespoons coconut sugar
- 4 tablespoons plus 1/2 almond flour
- pinch of pink low of sodium salt
- 1 cup canned coconut cream/milk, full fat, room temperature
- 1/2 teaspoon vanilla

CUPCAKES

Ingredients:

- 1 1/2 cups fine blanched almond flour
- 1 1/2 teaspoons baking powder
- 1/2 teaspoon pink low sodium salt
- 1/2 cup canned coconut cream/milk, full fat, room temperature
- 2 tablespoons unsalted grass-fed butter, plus more for greasing
- 2 organic cage-free eggs
- 1 cup coconut palm sugar
- 1 teaspoon vanilla

CHOCOLATE GANACHE

Ingredients:

- 1 cup Mini Chocolate Chips
- 1/4 cup canned coconut cream/milk, full fat, room temperature
- 4 tablespoons unsalted grass-fed butter
- 1 teaspoon vanilla

Instructions:

- Start by making the Vanilla Cream. In a small bowl whisk egg yolks together until smooth, set aside. In a medium saucepan combine stevia, coconut palm sugar, arrowroot, and salt and stir over medium heat. Add milk in a slow steady stream. Stir and let cook until the mixture begins to boil and thicken, about 5 minutes.

- Pour 1/3 of the milk mixture into the yolks and stir together with a whisk until combined. Then pour back into the saucepan with the rest of the milk mixture and cook over medium heat, stirring often, until thick, about 3 minutes. Now stir in the vanilla.

- Use a fine sieve to pour the vanilla mixture through into a small bowl. Cover it with plastic wrap and press the wrap down directly onto the surface of the cream. Refrigerate until very cold, an hour at least. While you wait, prepare your cupcakes and chocolate ganache.

- Preheat the oven to 350 degrees. Grease a mini cupcake pan very liberally with butter. In a large bowl combine almond flour, baking powder and salt, use a fork to stir together. Warm coconut cream/milk and butter in a saucepan over low heat.

- In a separate large bowl, whisk together eggs and coconut palm sugar. Then fold in the dry mixture. Bring the coconut cream/milk and butter mixture to a boil. Add this mixture to the batter and whisk until smooth. Now stir in the vanilla. Pour batter into a Ziploc bag, cut a small hole in the corner. Transfer batter to prepared pan, filling to the top. Bake for 10-12 minutes or until a toothpick comes out clean. While you are waiting for the cupcakes to cool, go ahead and make your chocolate ganache.

- Using the double boiler method, melt together the chocolate, coconut cream/milk and butter. Once melted and combined, stir in the vanilla.

- Transfer ganache to a Ziploc bag once it's cool enough, and cut a small hole in the corner tip.

- Once your cupcakes are cool, remove two from the pan at a time. Squeeze a layer of vanilla cream over the top of one cupcake and then flip the other one upside down and use it to sandwich the two together. Then pour your chocolate ganache over the top and enjoy!

VANILLA CUPCAKES WITH MOCHA CREAM

Ingredients

For the cupcakes
- 1/4 cup coconut flour
- 1/4 teaspoon low sodium salt
- 1/8 teaspoon baking soda
- Seeds scraped from half a vanilla bean
- 1/2 teaspoon vanilla extract
- 2 large eggs
- 1/4 cup coconut oil
- 2 drops stevia liquid

For the frosting:
- 4 tablespoons butter, at room temperature
- 9 drops stevia liquid
- 1 tablespoon cocoa
- Tiny pinch of low sodium salt
- 1/4 teaspoon vanilla extract
- 1/4 teaspoon finely ground coffee
- Coffee beans for garnish

Instructions

- Preheat the oven to 350 and line a muffin tin with paper liners.

- Whisk together the coconut flour, salt, and baking soda in a medium bowl. Add the vanilla bean seeds, and mix together with your fingers, pinching the mixture to evenly distribute the vanilla seeds.

- In a small bowl, whisk together the vanilla extract, eggs, coconut oil, and stevia. Add the wet ingredients to the dry and whisk well, or beat with a hand mixer, until very smooth.

- Pour the batter into the cupcake cups and bake for 15-20 minutes, or until a toothpick comes out clean.

- Using a hand mixer, beat the butter until very smooth. Add the remaining ingredients and beat until incorporated. If your frosting does not seem stiff enough, refrigerate for a little while, then beat again.

- Once the cupcakes are completely cool, pipe or spread on the frosting . Top with a coffee bean if desired.

MEATY MEATLOAF CUPCAKES

Ingredients

- 2 lbs of lean ground beef
- 4 eggs
- 2 cups almond flour
- 1 teaspoon dried basil
- 1 teaspoon garlic powder
- 1 medium onion
- 2 tablespoons Worcestershire sauce
- Salt and pepper to taste
- 5-6 sweet potatoes
- 1/2 cup butter or coconut oil
- 1 teaspoon Salt

Instructions

- Preheat the oven to 375 degrees. Finely dice the onion or puree in a blender or food processor.
- In a large bowl, combine the meat, eggs, flour, basil, garlic powder, pureed onion, Worcestershire sauce, and salt and pepper and mix by hand until incorporated.
- Grease a muffin tin with coconut oil or butter and evenly divide the mixture into the muffin tins to make 2-3 meat "muffins" per person. If you don't have a muffin tin, you can just press the mixture into the bottom of a baking dish.
- Put into oven on middle rack, and put a baking

sheet with a rim under it, in case the oil from the meat happens to spill over

- For sweet potatoes: if they are small enough, you can put them into the oven at the same time, if not you can peel, cube and boil them until soft.

- When the meat is almost done, make sure sweet potatoes are cooked by whichever method you prefer, and drain the water if you boil them.

- Mix with butter and salt or pepper if desired and mash by hand or with an immersion blender.

- Remove meat "muffins" from the oven when they are cooked through

and remove from the tin. Top each with a dollop of the mashed sweet potatoes to make it look like a cupcake.

GUAVA CUPCAKES

Ingredients

Cake

- 1 cup of Coconut Flour
- 1 cup almond Flour
- 1/4 cup of Light Olive Oil
- 4 Tablespoons Coconut Sugar
- 5 drops stevia liquid
- 1 cup of Concentrated Guava Puree
- 3 Eggs
- 1 teaspoon of Lime Juice

- 1 teaspoon of Cream of Tartar
- 1 teaspoon of Baking Soda
- teaspoon of Salt

Whipped Guava Frosting
- 1 cup of room temperature coconut oil
- 5 Tablespoons of Concentrated Guava Puree
- 7 drops stevia liquid
- 1 cup of almond flour
- 1 teaspoon of Lime

Instructions

- You may have to boil the guava puree until the applesauce is thick.
- Preheat the oven to 350 F. We will drop the temperature to 325 F to bake. Line the muffin tin with cupcake liners. Separate the eggs into egg yolks and egg whites.
- Combine the egg whites and cream of tartar and beat with a whisk attachment on high speed. Place the whites in a bowl and set aside, or store in the refrigerator while preparing the rest of the ingredients. Combine the olive oil, egg yolks, stevia,

lime juice, and guava puree in the mixing bowl and beat on high speed for about 30 seconds.

- Sift together the coconut flour, tapioca flour, baking soda, sugar, and salt to make the dry flour mixture.

- Add half of the dry flour mixture to the wet mixture and whip until the flours absorb and the batter becomes fluffy. Scrape the sides with a spatula to incorporate.

- Add the rest of the dry flour mixture and beat on high speed with the whisk until combined and fluffy.

- Scoop in a heaping of the egg white meringue and hand mix into the batter. Gently fold in the rest of the meringue until combined.

- Portion the batter into each cake pan and place tin in the oven centered.

- Reduce the temperature to 325 F and bake for 25-30 minutes until an inserted toothpick comes out clean.

- Let cool to room temperature or colder before frosting. Chill the beaters and mixing bowl in the freezer for about 15 minutes.

- Combine the raw stevia and guava puree in a cup until it forms a thicker syrup.

- Whip the coconut shortening and optionally the

cream cheese. Add the arrowroot starch and salt and whip.

- While mixing on medium speed, pour the guava mixture slowly. Whip until pink.

BLUEBERRY MUFFINS

Ingredients

- 1/2 cups almond flour
- 1 Tablespoon coconut flour
- 1/4 teaspoon low sodium salt
- 1/2 teaspoon baking soda
- 1 Tablespoon vanilla
- 1/4 cup coconut oil
- 10 drops stevia liquid
- 1/4 cup coconut milk
- 2 eggs
- 1 cup fresh or frozen blueberries
- 2-3 Tablespoons cinnamon

Instructions

- Preheat the oven to 350 degrees. Line a 12 count muffin tin and lightly oil with coconut oil.

- In a mixing bowl combine almond flour, coconut flour, salt, and baking soda and stir to combine.

- Pour in coconut oil, eggs, stevia, coconut milk, and vanilla; mix well.

- Fold in blueberries and add cinnamon. Distribute into muffin tin. Sprinkle with additional cinnamon.
- Bake for 22-25 minutes. Allow to cool and enjoy!

CARROT GINGER MUFFINS

Ingredients:
- 2 cups blanched almond flour
- 1 teaspoon salt
- 1 teaspoon baking soda
- 1 tsp allspice
- 1 tsp powdered ginger
- a pinch of clove
- 1 cup shredded coconut shreds, unsweetened
- 2 eggs, preferably pastured
- 1/4 cup coconut oil, melted
- 20 drops stevia liquid
- 1-2 Tbsp grated fresh ginger
- 1 cup grated carrot
- 3/4 cup raisins, soaked in water for 15 minutes and drained

Instructions:
- In a large bowl, combine almond flour, salt, baking soda, spices, and coconut shreds
- In a smaller bowl whisk together eggs, oil, and syrup. Add fresh ginger, grated carrot, and raisins.

- Stir wet ingredients into dry; Spoon batter into paper-lined muffin tins

- Bake at 350° for 18-20 minutes for mini muffins OR 24-26 minutes for regular muffins.

PECAN MUFFINS

Ingredients
- 1/3 cup coconut flour
- 1/4 cup butter, melted
- 2 large eggs
- 1/3 cup chopped pecans
- 1/4 tsp baking powder stevia drops to taste

Instructions

- Whisk together the butter, eggs and molasses.Sieve the coconut flour and baking powder into a large mixing bowl.
- Gradually add the wet ingredients to the dry, stirring until it forms a thick, runny batter .

- Fold in the pecans.Spoon about a tbsp into small muffin cups.

- Bake at 350F for 10-12 minutes.

PERFECT PIZZA MUFFINS

Ingredients:

- 2 cups almond flour
- 4 eggs
- 1 cup coconut flour
- 1 cup melted coconut oil
- 1 tablespoon garlic powder
- 1 tablespoon parsley
- 1 tablespoon oregano
- 2 links of Italian sausage, finely chopped
- 3 slices of cooked bacon, finely chopped
- 1 cup spinach, finely chopped

INSTRUCTIONS

- Preheat the oven to 375 degrees.
- Mix all of the ingredients together, then scoop into the muffin tin. Fill each tin all the way to the top.
- Bake for about 30-45 minutes, or until firm.

SWEET POTATO MUFFINS

Ingredients:

- 1/2 cup Coconut Flour
- 2 Eggs
- 1 tsp Vanilla
- 1 tsp Salt
- 1 tsp Baking Soda

- 1 tsp Cinnamon
- 1/2 cup Ground Flax seed
- 2 Sweet Potatoes, baked and mashed
- 1 cup Raisins or Chocolate Chips (optional)

Instructions:

- Whisk together all the dry ingredients.

- Beat the eggs and add dry mix with spoonfuls until well blended.

- Add the mashed sweet potatoes. Spoon batter into lined muffin cups.

- Bake at 350 degrees for 30-35 minutes.

ZESTY ZUCCHINI MUFFINS

Ingredients

- 3/4 Cup applesauce
- 6 drops stevia liquid (May need a few more)
- 1/4 cup coconut oil, melted
- 3 eggs
- 1 Tbsp vanilla
- 1 Cup almond flour
- 1 1/2 tsp baking soda
- 1 Cup zucchini, shredded
- 3/4 Cup raisin

Instructions

- With electric or stand mixer, beat applesauce, stevia and oil

- Add eggs and vanilla and mix until combined

- Slowly mix in almond flour and soda, then beat until batter forms Fold in zucchini and raisins

- Bake at 350 degrees for 25 minutes.

COZY COCONUT MUFFINS
Ingredients
- 1/2 cup coconut flour
- 2 eggs, at room temperature
- 1 cup almond milk
- 1 tsp stevia
- 1 Tbsp coconut oil
- 1 Tbsp coconut milk at room temperature
- 2 tsp. vanilla extract
- 1/4 tsp. baking soda
- 1 tsp. apple cider vinegar

Instructions

- Preheat the oven to 350 degrees and prepare a muffin tin with 8 liners.

- Combine the coconut flour and eggs until smooth. Add the remaining ingredients and stir well.

- Divide evenly between the muffin tins. Bake until golden and a toothpick comes out clean, about 20 minutes.

LEMON MOUSSE CUPCAKES

Ingredients:
- 1/2 cup coconut flour
- 2 eggs, at room temperature
- 1 tsp stevia
- 1 Tbsp coconut oil
- 2 Tbsp coconut milk at room temperature
- 1 tsp. vanilla extract
- 1/2 tsp. ground cardamom
- 1/4 tsp. baking soda
- 1/2 tsp. apple cider vinegar

Lemon Mousse Frosting
- 2 oz cream cheese
- 8 tbsp heavy whipping cream
- 2 Tbsp butter
- 4 tbsp almond milk
- 8 tbsp powdered erythritol
- 1 tbsp lemon zest

Instructions:

- Preheat the oven to 350 degrees and prepare a muffin tin with 8 liners.

- Combine the coconut flour and eggs until smooth. Add the remaining ingredients and stir well.

- Divide evenly between the muffin tins. Bake for 20 minutes. Allow to cool completely and frost with the lemon mousse.

SAVORY MUFFINS

Ingredients

- 1 cup coconut flour
- 1 tsp baking soda
- 2-1 tsp low sodium salt
- 1/2 cup coconut oil
- cup + 2 tbsp coconut milk
- 3 pastured eggs
- 1 tsp apple cider vinegar
- 1 tsp garlic powder
- tsp each of rosemary, thyme, sage

Instructions

- Preheat the oven to 350°F. Melt the coconut oil and combine with remaining muffin ingredients in a food processor or bowl, mix well.

- Place batter in a muffin tin lined with muffin liners. The muffins will raise a small amount, so you can fill the muffin liner about half full-almost to the top.

- Bake for about 20-30 minutes or until a toothpick inserted comes out clean and the tops are slightly browned.

- Let it cool and slice in small squares.

MOLTEN LAVA CHOCOLATE CUPCAKE

- 4 oz Bittersweet chocolate
- 1 tsp Vanilla Extract
- 1/8 tsp Salt
- 7 drops stevia
- 2 tsp Coconut Flour
- 1 tsp Cacao Powder
- 2 eggs
- 1 Tbsp coconut oil

Instructions:

- Preheat the oven to 375 F. Grease four 6 oz ramekins with coconut oil.

- In a 4 cup measuring cup or medium microwave-safe bowl, melt chocolate and coconut oil in the microwave on low power. Stir until smooth and let cool.

- In a small bowl, beat eggs, vanilla, salt and sugar with a hand mixer until light and frothy, about five minutes.

- Pour egg mixture over chocolate. Sift cocoa and

coconut flour over the top. Then gently fold all the ingredients together.

- Pour batter into prepared ramekins (they should be filled to within the top).

- Place the ramekins on a baking sheet and place in the oven (you can chill the ramekins for a few hours if you want to make them ahead of time, just make sure you bring them back to room temperature before baking). Bake for 11-12 minutes. Remove from the oven and serve immediately.

CARROT CUPCAKES

Ingredients:

- 2 eggs
- 1 tablespoon non-dairy milk
- 1 tablespoon coconut oil
- 1 tablespoon carrot juice
- 2 tablespoon egg whites
- 10 drops liquid stevia
- 1 teaspoon pure vanilla extract
- 7 tablespoon coconut flour
- 1 teaspoon baking powder
- pinch ground cinnamon

Instructions

- Preheat the oven to 350 F and line 12 muffin tins with medium-sized paper liners.
- Place eggs and egg white in a blender and beat well, about 30 seconds.
- Pour in carrot juice, milk, coconut oil, stevia and vanilla. Blend quickly to mix.
- Drop in dry ingredients and mix for about 10 seconds. Pour into prepared muffin tins and bake for 25-30 minutes.
- Remove from the pan and allow to cool on the cooling rack for at least 1 hour before applying buttercream.

CINNAMON CHOCOLATE CHIP MUFFINS

Ingredients

- 2 large eggs
- 5 drops stevia liquid
- 1 teaspoon vanilla extract
- 4 tablespoons unsalted butter, melted
- 3/4 cup coconut flour
- 1 tablespoon ground cinnamon
- 2 teaspoons baking powder
- 1 teaspoon baking soda
- small pinch salt

Instructions

- Preheat oven to 375 f and adjust rack to middle position .Line with muffin liners
- Whisk eggs, stevia, vanilla, butter, and applesauce in a large mixing bowl or use a stand mixer
- Sift coconut flour, cinnamon, baking powder, baking soda, and salt over a medium bowl
- Add dry ingredients to wet ingredients and until well blended
- Fold in chocolate chips ensuring an even distribution throughout your batter
- Spoon batter into muffin cups and bake for 16-18 minutes.Remove the muffins from the oven and let cool.

STRAWBERRY SHORTCAKE CUPCAKES

Ingredients:
- 2 cups blanched almond flour
- 1 teaspoon baking soda
- 5 drops stevia liquid
- 1 cup coconut oil, melted
- 2 large eggs, room temperature
- 1 tablespoon lemon juice
- 2 teaspoons vanilla extract
- 1 teaspoon lemon zest
- 1 cup finely chopped strawberries

Frosting
- 2 egg whites, room temperature
- drops stevia liquid
- 1 teaspoon lemon juice or vinegar
- 1 tablespoons strawberry preserves

Instructions:
- Preheat the oven to 325 F. Line a standard muffin tin with baking cups.

- Combine the stevia, coconut oil, eggs, lemon juice, vanilla, and lemon zest in the jar of a blender. Puree on medium speed for 20 seconds or until frothy and smooth.

- Add the dry ingredients and blend on high for 30-45 seconds. The batter should be very smooth and contain no lumps.

- Gently fold the chopped strawberries in by hand. Divide the batter evenly into the muffin tin, filling about half of the way full.

- Bake for 16-18 minutes, until a toothpick can be inserted into the middle and comes out clean.

- Let the cupcakes cool completely on the counter before frosting. Once the cupcakes have cooled, make your Italian meringue.

- Bring your stevia to a boil in a saucepan over medium-high heat.

- Meanwhile, beat the egg whites and lemon juice until frothy and you can just begin to see trail marks from your beaters. When you lift out the beaters, you should see soft peaks.

- With the beaters or mixer running, slowly pour in the boiling stevia in a steady stream. Continue beating for 6-8 minutes, until the meringue is cool to the touch.

- Gently fold in the strawberry preserves. Put the frosting into a piping bag for a pretty design, or spread onto cupcakes with a knife.

BREAKFAST CUPCAKES

Ingredients

- 1/3 cup mashed sweet potato
- 2 eggs
- 5 drops stevia liquid
- 1 teaspoon pure vanilla extract
- 1 cup grated carrot
- 1 cup grated apple
- 2 teaspoons fresh ginger, peeled and grated, optional
- 2 cups blanched almond flour
- 1 cup unsweetened shredded coconut
- 2/3 cup raisins
- 2/3 cup raw walnuts, chopped
- 2 teaspoons ground cinnamon
- 1 teaspoon baking powder
- 1 teaspoon baking soda
- 1 teaspoon salt

Instructions

- Preheat the oven to 350 degrees F and line a 12-cupcake tray with baking cups.

- Whisk together the mashed sweet potato, eggs, stevia, grated carrot, apple, and ginger until well-combined (wet ingredients).

- In a separate mixing bowl, stir together the almond flour, raisins, walnuts, cinnamon, baking powder, baking soda, and salt (dry ingredients).

Pour the dry mixture into the bowl with the wet mixture and stir well until a thick batter forms.

- using an ice cream scoop or small measuring cup, scoop batter into the lined muffin tray, filling the cups 3/4 of the way up.

- Place the cupcake tray on the center rack in the preheated oven and bake for 30 to 35 minutes, until cupcake tests clean when poked with a toothpick.

COFFEE CUPCAKES

Ingredients:
- 4 eggs
- 1/4 cup ghee
- 1/4 cup coconut flour
- 1/4 cup water chestnut flour
- 1 Tbsp vanilla
- 6 drops stevia liquid
- 1/2 tsp cinnamon

Topping
- 1/2 cup chopped pecans
- 5 drops stevia liquid
- 1 Tbsp ghee
- 2 tsp instant coffee
- 2 Tbsp almond flour
- 1 tsp cinnamon

Instructions

- Preheat the oven to 350 degrees. Put eggs in a large mixing bowl and mix thoroughly with an immersion blender until frothy.

- Add remaining ingredients and mix well. Fill the muffin pan evenly .Place in the oven and set the timer for 20 minutes. Now combine ingredients for the topping in a separate bowl.

- At the 20 minute mark take out the muffins and add the topping evenly between all the muffins. Put them back in the oven for another 10 minutes. Broil for an additional 2 minutes and remove quickly.

LEMON POPPY SEED CUPCAKE

Ingredients

- 1/4 cup almond flour
- 2 tbsp coconut flour
- 1 tbsp poppy seeds
- 1 tsp baking soda
- 1 tsp baking powder
- 1/4 tsp low sodium salt
- 3 drops stevia liquid
- 1/4 cup fresh lemon juice, plus the zest of 1 lemon
- 2 eggs whisked
- 1 tsp vanilla extract

Instructions

- Preheat the oven to 350-degrees F. In a small bowl, mix all the wet ingredients together.

- In a bowl, combine all the dry ingredients. Now pour the wet ingredients into the dry ingredients bowl, and stir into a batter.

- Let the batter set for a few minutes, then stir it again.

- Grease a muffin tin or use muffin liners and fill each well or cup about two-thirds full.
- Bake about 15-20 minutes, or until a toothpick inserted into a muffin comes out clean

STRAWBERRY CHIA CUPCAKE

Ingredients
- 1 cup + 2 tbsp coconut flour
- 1 tsp xanthan gum
- 1 tsp baking powder
- 1 tsp baking soda
- 1 tbsp chia seeds
- 1 tbsp lemon zest
- 1 tbsp coconut oil
- 1 large egg, room temperature
- 1 tsp vanilla extract
- 1 cup Greek yogurt
- 1 cup agave
- 1 tbsp freshly squeezed lemon juice
- 1 cup vanilla almond milk
- 2 scoops vanilla protein powder
- 1 cup strawberries

Instructions
- Preheat the oven to 350°F, and lightly coat 9 standard-sized muffin cups with nonstick cooking spray.

- Whisk together the coconut flour, xanthan gum, baking powder, baking soda, salt, chia seeds, and lemon zest in a medium bowl. In a separate bowl, whisk together the coconut oil or butter, egg, and vanilla. Stir in the Greek yogurt until no large lumps remain. Stir in the agave, lemon juice, and almond milk. Mix in the protein powder.

- Add in the coconut flour mixture, stirring until fully incorporated. Let the batter rest for 10 minutes. Gently fold in the diced strawberries

- Divide the batter between the prepared muffin cups. Bake at 350°F for 2528 minutes, or until a toothpick inserted into the center comes out clean. Cool in the pan for 10 minutes before carefully turning out onto a wire rack.

TRIPLE COCONUT CUPCAKES

Ingredients
- 1 cup almond flour
- 3 tbsp coconut flour
- 1 cup shredded coconut
- 2 tsp baking powder
- 6 drops stevia liquid
- 2 eggs, separated
- 1/4 cup coconut oil
- 1 tbsp vanilla extract

Instructions
- Preheat the oven to 350 F. Grease a muffin tin or line with muffin cups.
- Combine almond flour, coconut flour, shredded coconut, salt and baking powder in a medium mixing bowl.

- Mix the egg yolks, stevia, coconut oil and vanilla

extract in a small mixing bowl. Add to the almond flour mixture and combine thoroughly.

- Using a hand mixer, whip the egg whites until they form stiff peaks.

- Stir the egg whites into the rest of the ingredients, spoon the batter into the muffin tin.

- Bake for 25 minutes (or until the tops are nicely browned and a tester comes out clean.

LEMON-COCONUT MUFFINS

Ingredients
- 1/4 cup almond flour
- 2 tbsp coconut oil
- 1 tsp vanilla extract
- 1 cup shredded unsweetened coconut
- 1tbs coconut flour
- 1/2 tsp baking soda
- 1/2 tsp baking powder
- 1/4 tsp low sodium salt
- 5 drops stevia liquid
- 1/3 cup fresh lemon juice, plus the zest of 1 lemon
- 1/4 cup full-fat coconut milk
- 2 eggs

Instructions

- Preheat the oven to 350° F. In a small bowl, mix all the wet ingredients together. In a medium bowl, combine all the dry ingredients.
- Now pour the wet ingredients into the dry ingredients bowl, and stir into a batter. Let the batter set for a few minutes, then stir it again. Grease a muffin tin or use silicone muffin liners and fill each well or cup about two-thirds full. Bake for about 18-23 minutes.

CHOCOLATE BANANA MUFFINS

Ingredients
- 2 medium ripe bananas
- 5 drops stevia liquid
- 1 teaspoon vanilla extract
- 2 eggs
- 1/4 cup coconut oil
- 2 cups blanched almond flour
- 3 tablespoons coconut flour
- 1/3 cup cocoa powder
- 1 teaspoon baking soda
- 1 cup semi-sweet chocolate chips
- Additional mini chocolate chips for sprinkling, if desired

Instructions

- Preheat the oven to 350°F and line a muffin tin with 12 muffin liners.In a large bowl, mash the bananas with the bottom of a glass. They should almost be like a puree.Add the stevia and vanilla and stir.

- Add in the eggs and oil and stir until well combined.In a medium bowl, mix together the almond flour, coconut flour, cocoa powder, baking soda and salt.

- Stir just until combined and then stir in the chocolate chips.Spoon the batter into the muffin liners and sprinkle on additional chocolate chips, if desired. Bake for 18 minutes or until a toothpick inserted in the center comes out clean.

ENGLISH CUPCAKES

Ingredients:

- 1 cup almond flour
- 1 tablespoon coconut flour
- 1 teaspoon baking soda 1 teaspoon salt
- 1 egg
- 1 tablespoon coconut oil
- 2 tablespoons water
- 1/2 teaspoon cinnamon
- 5 drops stevia liquid
- 1 tablespoons golden raisins

Instructions:

- Whisk together the dry ingredients in a small bowl.
- Add the remaining wet ingredients and whisk again until fully incorporated. Transfer the mixture into a greased microwave safe ramekin. Microwave for 2 minutes.
- Remove from the ramekin, slice the muffin in half and toast for 2-3 minutes in a toaster oven.
- Serve with softened butter.

ALMOND FLOUR CUPCAKES

Ingredients:
- 2-1/2 cups almond flour or almond meal
- 1 tsp baking soda
- 1 tsp low sodium salt
- 2 large eggs
- 1 cup unsweetened (pumpkin puree, apple sauce, or mashed banana)
- 3 drops stevia, agave nectar or stevia
- 2 tablespoons melted coconut oil
- 1 teaspoon vinegar
- Optional Flavorings: 1 teaspoon extract (e.g., vanilla, almond), citrus zest, dried herbs (e.g., basil, dill), or spice (e.g., cinnamon, cumin)
- 1 cup fresh fruit (blueberries, diced apple) or cup dried fruit/cacao nibs/chopped nuts

Instructions:
- Preheat the oven to 350 F. Line 10 cups in a standard 12-cup muffin tin with paper or foil liners.

- In a large bowl whisk the almond flour, baking soda and salt (whisk in any dried spices or herbs at this point, if using).

- In a small bowl, whisk the eggs, pumpkin, stevia, oil and vinegar (add any extracts or zest at this point, if using).

- Add the wet ingredients to the dry ingredients, stirring until blended. Fold in any optional stir-ins, if using. Divide batter evenly among prepared cups.

- Bake in a preheated oven for 14 to 18 minutes until set at the centers and golden brown at the edges.

DELIGHTFUL CINNAMON APPLE MUFFINS

Ingredients:
- 1 cup unsweetened applesauce
- 2 eggs
- 1/4 cup coconut oil, melted
- 1 tsp vanilla
- Stevia to taste
- 1/2 cup coconut flour
- 1 tsp cinnamon
- 1 tsp baking powder
- 1 tsp baking soda
- 1/4 tsp salt

Instructions:

- Preheat the oven to 350 F. Line a muffin tin with liners. In a large bowl, add applesauce, eggs, coconut oil, stevia, and vanilla. Stir to combine.

- Stir in the coconut flour, cinnamon, baking powder, baking soda, and low sodium salt. Distribute the batter evenly into the lined muffin tins, filling each about two-thirds of the way full.

- Bake for 15-20 minutes, until a toothpick inserted into the center comes out clean.

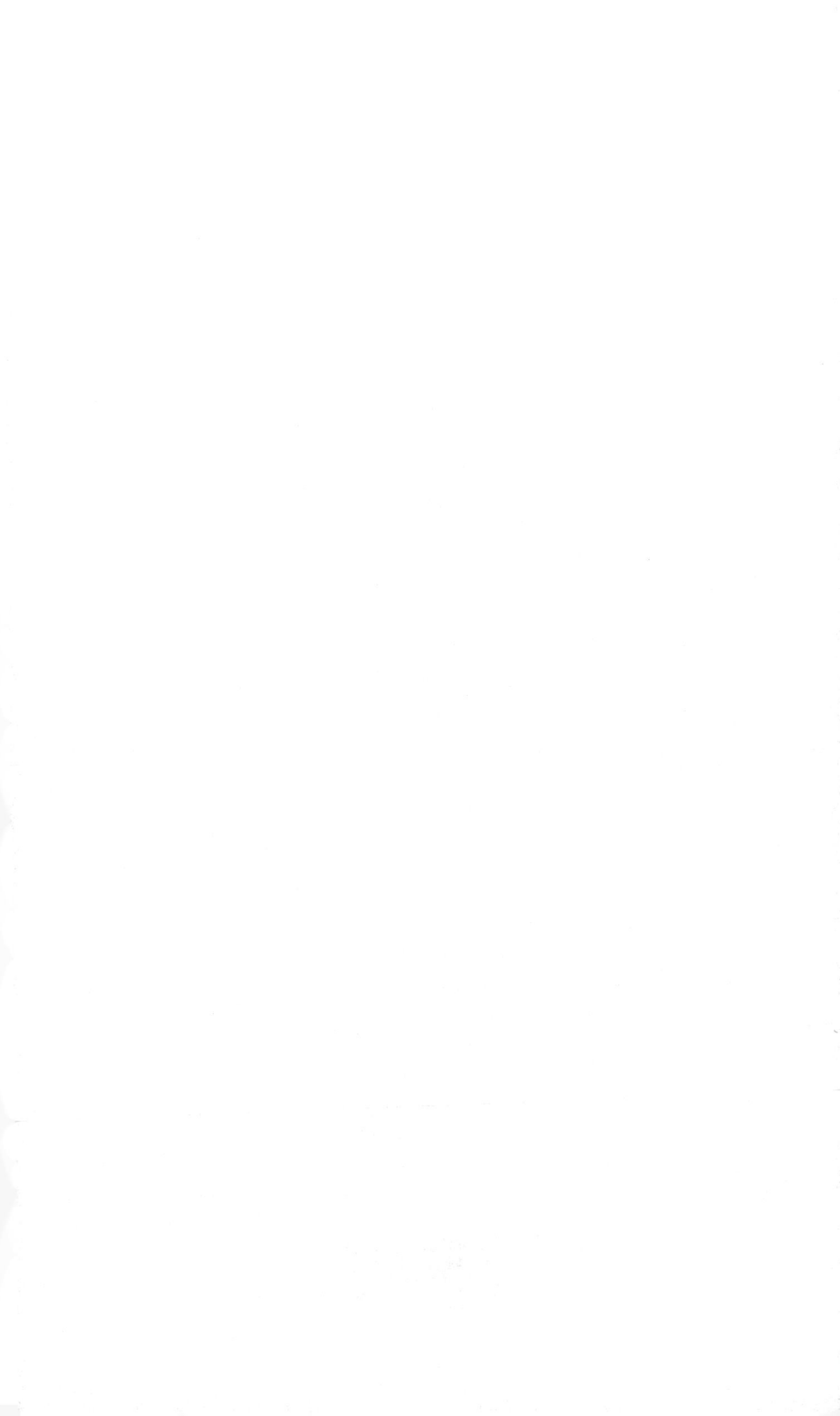

Made in the USA
Monee, IL
07 May 2023